53 Ways

TO USE
NONI FRUIT JUICE
For Your Better Health

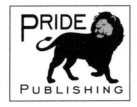

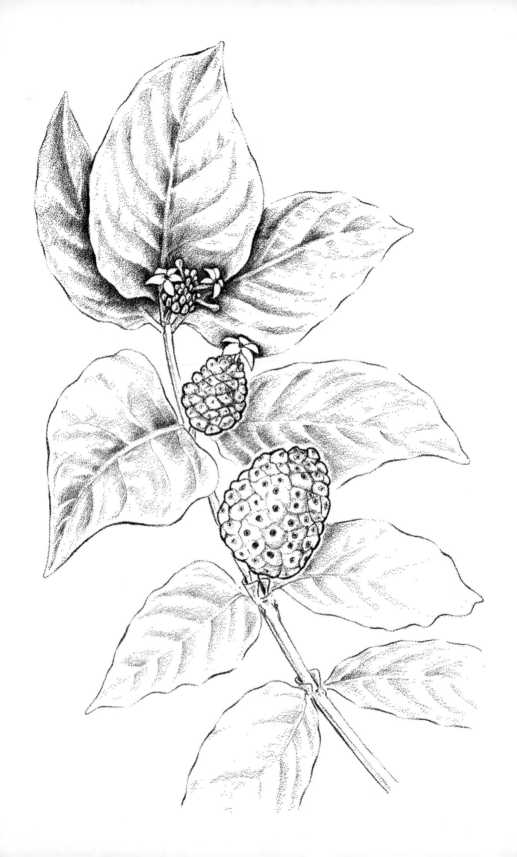

PRAISE FOR:
53 WAYS TO USE NONI FRUIT JUICE

"Isabelle Navarre-Brown has done a masterful job. *53 Ways to Use Noni Fruit Juice* is certain to help the newcomer as well as the long-time user of Noni fruit juice in showing the myriad uses for this amazing product."

– Donald J. Mantell, M.D.

"This book answered many of the questions that people are continually asking us about how to use the Noni fruit juice for various applications. We found it very insightful and quite informative. We feel that anyone who uses the Noni would benefit from a thorough reading of *53 Ways to Use Noni Fruit Juice*. It is now kept in our medical reference library to be used as the need arises. We would suggest that any believer in the healing properties of the Noni plant do the same."

– Floyd and Ann Holdman

"When I first started taking Noni, it cleared my arthritis. But after a while, the pain returned. Then I tried one of the techniques in this book—Interrupting Noni Therapy—and it worked! Noni is now helping my arthritis better than before. Besides being an arsenal of tools for using Noni, *53 Ways to Use Noni* is an excellent marketing tool, and I would recommend that everyone have a copy."

– Sal Serio

"*53 Ways to Use Noni* is a fascinating book. It provides simple, easy to use techniques for using Noni in almost every situation. The remedy for tooth aches and the Headache Compress have done wonders for my family, and my 4 year old son who is a diabetic takes Noni regularly. Not only did we try the ideas for giving Noni to children, but we also tell Josh he will get muscles like the man on the front of the bottle and that has done wonders! He calls Noni his "muscle juice" and compares himself to the man with every dose. I also noticed amazing results when I gave Josh the Noni before every meal rather than just a morning dose. The suggestions in this book for using Noni fruit juice for diabetes really have made a difference!
"This book is exactly what the world needs, with helpful remedies in an easy to read format. Now Noni users everywhere can experience the miraculous benefits from Noni in more ways than just taking a daily dose. Isa has done an incredible job introducing Noni and its benefits to the world."

–Emily Freeman

By the same author:

42 WAYS TO USE NONI
SKIN LOTION
A HANDBOOK OF TOPICAL APPLICATIONS

HEALING SECRETS OF NONI
A PRACTICAL GUIDE TO NONI DILUTIONS
AND HARMONICS

53 Ways

TO USE
NONI FRUIT JUICE
For Your Better Health

A HANDBOOK OF ORAL, TOPICAL
AND INTERNAL APPLICATIONS AND PROCEDURES

ISABELLE NAVARRE-BROWN

Pride Publishing
500 South Geneva Road
Vineyard, Utah 84058

53 Ways to Use Noni Fruit Juice for Your Better Health
A Handbook of Oral, Topical and Internal
Applications & Procedures

Illustrated by Valerie Mortensen.
Edited by Emily Freeman and Stephen Navarre-Brown.
Back cover photo by Napoletano Studio.
Cover Design by Robert Evelyn Design Group.
Printed in the United States of America.
ISBN 1-887938-21-4

Second Edition

– IMPORTANT NOTICE –

The information in this book is designed to provide health
information for purposes of reference and guidance and to
accompany, not replace, the services of a qualified health care
practitioner or physician. It is not the intent of the author or
publisher to prescribe any substance to cure, mitigate, treat,
or prevent any disease. In the event you use this information
with or without seeking medical attention, the author and
publisher shall not be liable or otherwise responsible for any
loss, damage or injury caused or arising out of, directly or indirectly, by the information contained in this book or its use.

DEDICATION

Our daughter was born two weeks after we started taking
Noni fruit juice. The idea for this book came soon after. We felt
it was very significant that these three events happened so
closely together.

In ancient Polynesia, a family's knowledge of healing was
compiled and passed from one generation to the next. Though
we have published this information so that others may benefit,
this book is our family's collection of knowledge about Noni.

In following the Polynesian tradition, I pass this knowledge
to our daughter, Aria Ray, as I dedicate this book to her.

CONTENTS

CONTENTS

ACKNOWLEDGEMENTS

In thinking about the many who supported and contributed to this book, my gratitude must go first to Nature herself, for developing the remarkable *Morinda citrifolia*, or Noni plant, and then to generations of Polynesians whose use of the Noni fruit left the world a powerful legacy.

May I also take this opportunity to personally thank Mitchell Tate for "finding" Noni and bringing it to the attention of John Wadsworth and Stephen Story who made Noni palatable for modern tastebuds. Thank you also to Kerry Asay, Kim Asay and Kelly Olsen for their untiring effort to help bring Noni fruit juice to the world, and to the President of French Polynesia, Mssr. Gaston Floss, and the Country's Vice-President, Mssr. Edouard Fritch, for their generous support of Noni agriculture and export. Many thanks are also due Dr. Annie Hirazumi, Dr. Ralph Heinicke, Dr. Charles Garnier, and researchers of Noni around the world for their efforts and inspiration to examine Noni scientifically.

Our friends and business associates also deserve a warm "thank you" for trying many of the techniques in this book and giving us their feedback. I wish to thank all of you, and in particular, Catherine Sarnoski, Dennis and Carol Kotopoulis, Don and Nancy Failla, Carol LaBarge, Tina Erwin, Glenn Raney,

xiii

Jay Coons, Dave Peacock, Kent Murphy, Bonnie and Bob Landino, Helen King, Ann Eckroth, Jodie Snyder, and Becky Yoder for her help with the Noni Colonic Irrigation, Dr. Don Mantell for his marvelous enthusiasm, and Dr. Ken Stejskal for his open-hearted anticipation of the book.

Special thanks also to our friends who agreed to review the manuscript and/or offer their feedback or endorsement: Floyd and Ann, Tom and Mannie, Ken and Mary, Sal and Joan, Del and Sylvia, and Dr. Bryant Bloss.

I am also very grateful to Dr. Ralph Heinicke for reviewing the manuscript and offering his feedback, and to Dr. Steven Hall for his review and feedback, and especially for writing the foreword to this book.

Thank you to Valerie, who drew the illustrations, to Emily for her editorial suggestions and endorsement, to Beth for getting me started on Photoshop®, to Mark for his help with MSWord®, Pagemaker® and all our computer questions, and to Mac and Colby for being so easy to work with. Thank you also to the Hair Gallery and Salon in Marlborough, Connecticut for supplying some of the hair samples that I used in my research for the Noni Scalp Treatment.

Like saving dessert for after dinner, I wait for the end of these acknowledgements to share my most loving gratitude. Indeed, my heart bursts when my thoughts turn to my husband, Stephen, and daughter, Aria Ray. They spent many an afternoon wandering through toystores so that I could have some quiet time at home to work on this book, and many an evening alone together during the final stages of this project. Surely, without Stephen and Aria's support, this book could not and would not have been written. Thank you my dear ones.

FOREWORD

During the first half of this Century, a great deal of common-sense health care information was lost as our country went through the institutionalization and industrialization of medicine. This resulted in large segments of the population putting their care (along with their personal choices and power) into the hands of physicians, pharmaceutical companies and technology. The second half of this Century, it seems, has been a reclaiming of our common-sense knowledge, personal choices and personal power. This process of reclamation has come in waves, each wave growing as new waves developed.

The first wave was a growing awareness of the importance of good foods, then came the wave of vitamins and minerals, then the wave of phytonutrients (antioxidants, alkaloids, glucopolysaccharides, etc.) and herbs. I believe that Noni fruit juice exemplifies the crest of this latest wave. Phytonutrients represent a step beyond what we traditionally call "vitamins". They are specialized plant compounds that have beneficial functions in our bodies. Examples of good sources of phytonutrients you may already be familiar with include ginseng, licorice, ginkgo biloba and aloe vera.

Noni fruit juice is known to contain many different kinds of phytonutrients. These include a glucopolysaccharide that is known to boost the immune system, a compound that inhibits viruses and cancerous changes in DNA, and the precursor to an alkaloid called xeronine that improves the functioning of your enzymes and cell wall receptors. These compounds work together to boost each other's effectiveness. And, they have been designed and formulated by the wisdom of nature rather than by someone in a laboratory. I have been working in the field of conventional, nutritional and alternative medicine for twelve years and I have not seen another natural substance as interesting and widely effective as Noni fruit juice.

Optimal functioning of your immune system is vital to your overall wellness, every biochemical reaction in your body utilizes enzymes and all of your cellular communication mechanisms use cell wall receptors. Because Noni fruit juice works on such basic levels, you can well imagine that it has many uses. And, indeed, this is what we see clinically. I have used Noni fruit juice in my practice since October, 1996, and have seen dramatic results in hundreds of people. I have talked with yet hundreds more from all around the Country who are also seeing dramatic results from Noni fruit juice.

The concept of Noni fruit juice is simple. It is just a juice. And it is as safe for you as orange juice or apple juice. So how could it have so many powerful therapeutic benefits? After all, in our pharmacological culture, don't powerful therapies belong in the domain of physicians and aren't they known to have powerful side-effects? Can't people hurt themselves with a powerful therapy if they don't know what they are doing?

Generally, yes, but think about it this way. If you were severely deficient in vitamin C, you would have a condition called scurvy. Vitamin C, among other things, helps with the production of collagen, the main ingredient in our connective tissue. So scurvy is a condition where your body is literally falling apart. If you had scurvy, a glass of orange juice would have powerful therapeutic benefits. A glass or two of orange juice per day would prevent it altogether, and you would have to drink a tremendous amount of orange juice to hurt yourself.

The analogy applies to Noni in that many of us are severely xeronine deficient. Nutrient-depleted soils, environmental pollution, the stress of everyday life, aging, diseases and certain food additives all work together to deplete our xeronine. Noni fruit juice supplies the necessary nutrients so that our bodies can make more xeronine.

As with other nutrients, herbs or remedies, the more you know about Noni fruit juice, the more you can obtain its full benefits. This is the power and beauty of this book—that it can help you understand the wide range of applications of Noni fruit juice. When I first read *53 Ways to Use Noni Fruit Juice*, even after a year of using Noni fruit juice myself and in my practice, many of the concepts and applications were new to me. And I have to admit, I was somewhat skeptical. But I tried some of the suggestions myself and recommended others to patients and watched what happened. Now I am a believer.

I think that Isabelle Navarre-Brown has successfully synthesized intuitive and experimental science to bring us this straightforward yet comprehensive guide to the many uses of Noni fruit juice. I expect that this book will help you receive even more benefit from this juice, this amazing gift from God.

Steven M. Hall, M.D.
January 5, 1998

xvii

WHAT YOU SHOULD KNOW ABOUT NONI FRUIT JUICE

There are several Noni fruit juice products on the market. Some are powdered and in capsules, and others are liquid. Of the liquid ones, some are the pure extract of the Noni fruit, and others are reconstituted from dried or powdered fruit. A few also contain extracts of the roots and leaves of the Noni plant.

In researching this book, I used juice that is a pure extract of the Noni fruit. It contains the perfect mix of the pulpy and the watery part of the fruit. This is important because these two fruit components, though essentially similar, have unique properties. Together, they are a dynamic pair.

I also feel it is important to know where the Noni that you use comes from. Noni grows in practically all tropical regions of the world, from Puerto Rico to India. However, the soils of the world simply aren't the same. The best Noni grows in unspoiled, nutrient rich soil—such as that of the remote Polynesian islands in the South Pacific. Juice from this

xix

compounds. Both these factors are critical to fully benefit from the applications in this book.

Please feel welcome to experiment with Noni fruit juice. Try a few of the procedures in this book. Customize them to suit your individual needs. Get to know Noni, by finding out how your body responds to different dosages. Which topical applications help you the most?

For us, Noni has become a life-long family friend. Read on, and allow me to introduce you...

INTRODUCTION

HOW MY EXPERIENCES
WITH NONI BEGAN:

"My cells remember this," I exclaimed moments after drinking my first ounce of Noni fruit juice. Somehow, Noni felt very familiar.

A few minutes later, changes started happening in my body. My heartburn subsided, I felt more calm and peaceful, and a tightness in my spine suddenly released. I was pregnant, and the premature labor contractions I was having never came back.

I suspected that Noni was special and began to experiment with it. Of all the nutritional supplements that had come to my attention over the years, nothing was as versatile and effective as Noni. I was amazed at all the ways that Noni proved helpful.

Generally, it is better to take Noni on an empty stomach. However, the Noni Anti-acid Substitute, which is taken after a meal, did wonders for my indigestion. I also used Noni Massage Oil to help prevent stretch-marks, and prepared Noni Tea to boost my immune system for the upcoming labor.

On October 30th, 1996, our daughter Aria Ray was born. My afterbirth cramps were very painful. Frequent Noni Compresses helped not only reduce the pain, but also heal the stitches I had received. A Trauma Dose sped my recovery, and a Maintenance Dose of two ounces a day helped me produce abundant milk to feed my baby.

Later, Noni Nose Drops cleared our infant's stuffy nose. The Noni Tummy Treatment helped her body overcome a fever, and the Noni Rash Plaster quickly took care of an occasional diaper rash.

One dose of Noni Ear Drops helped my husband's ear ache and the Topical Splash smoothed and softened his dry skin. The Noni Eye Poultice eased my eyestrain before my new eyeglasses arrived. And the Noni Small Area Treatment and First Aid for Minor Wounds has helped everyone in my family. We've been amazed at how quickly we have healed from cuts, scrapes, burns and scratches we've gotten from gardening, cooking, and caring for a large parrot.

OUR FAMILY'S MIRACLE:

In the summer of 1996, our German Shepherd dog, Aka, became severely ill. His hair fell out, and he scratched and chewed his body till it bled. Conventional treatment made him worse, and herbal and homeopathic remedies helped only a little.

In November, we tried giving him Noni. We followed the Procedure for Serious Conditions and every two weeks Interrupted Noni Therapy for a day or two. Twice a day we applied the Noni Topical Splash to his lesions. Five times a day, we used a plastic syringe to inject an ounce of Noni into his mouth.* He was very good about it. Maybe he knew it would help him feel better.

It did. By January he was completely healed. All his hair had grown back—in fact, it looked shinier and healthier than before. He also regained his playful joy for living.

Our whole family was so grateful for Noni!

---

* We used the 2:1 Dilution as described in my book *Healing Secrets of Noni.*

WHY NONI WORKS:

Although this book focuses on the myriad ways to use Noni, I wanted to touch on why Noni works. Researchers have identified over fifty compounds in the *Morinda citrifolia*, or Noni fruit, that have therapeutic value.[1]

Two of these compounds* have been proven to be helpful against bacteria, fungus, inflammation and allergies.[2] Another compound**, which is also found in essential oils, helps rejuvenate cells.[3] French scientists had success testing Noni's pain-killing elements.[4] Japanese researchers found a compound*** that inhibited pre-cancerous cells.[5] And Dr. Ralph Heinicke, of the University of Hawaii, discovered that Noni contains an appreciable quantity of a compound that he identified and named, "proxeronine".[6]

Proxeronine helps the body make an important alkaloid that Dr. Heinicke also discovered, which he called "xeronine". Xeronine is very important to the body because it regulates and strengthens the protein in our cells. Protein is found everywhere in our body, and does many things. For example, proteins comprise the bulk of the organic material within the cell. Hemoglobin, insulin, collagen, as well as muscle and skin, cell membranes, blood vessel walls, blood clots, and many hormones are also made of protein.[7] Xeronine's impact on protein may help to explain Noni's effectiveness for so many different conditions.[8]

If you would like to read more about Noni's ingredients and studies which have been done on Noni, may I suggest the books *Noni—Polynesia's Natural Pharmacy*,[9] and *Noni (Morinda citrifolia) Prize Herb of the South Pacific*.[10] Both are available from the company that distributes *53 Ways to Use Noni*.

---

*
Anthraquinones and scopoletin

**
Terpenes

***
Damnacanthal

xxiii

How to Use
This Book:

I have divided the fifty-three ways to use Noni fruit juice that are described in this book into three sections. Section 1 covers different ways to drink Noni. Section 2 describes topical uses, and Section 3 covers techniques for taking Noni internally.

Each of the fifty-three chapters in this book is also divided into three parts. In the first part, I suggest some conditions that a particular Noni application might help. This list is a guideline, and is not meant to provide medical advice or to be used as a prescription. If you have a condition that is not listed, but think the application might help, by all means try it. Of course, Noni won't always help everyone, even those who have conditions that are on the list.

In the second part of each chapter, I give detailed, step-by-step instructions on how to do each procedure. Third, I offer some helpful information about the procedure.

At the back of this book, you'll find four appendices that attempt to address some of the questions people most often ask us about Noni. The Health Evaluation Sheets in the first appendix are an invaluable tool for anyone looking to benefit from Noni. Appendix B contains information about cleansing reactions. Appendix C offers ideas why Noni may not work for you. Those who have found that Noni has stopped working for them may find some possible explanations in Appendix D. I am very grateful to Dr. Ralph Heinicke for offering some additional insights into this topic.

In this second edition I have made a few corrections to improve accuracy and readability. I have also added references to Noni Dilutions. Information about all fourteen Noni Dilutions, and their Harmonics, can be found in my book, *Healing Secrets of Noni.*

As you read this book, keep in mind that I am not a physician. The ideas that I offer for using Noni are not meant to replace your doctor's advice. I simply wanted to share what I know about Noni, and how my family has used Noni, so that you might have the opportunity to benefit as we have from this amazing and unique gift of nature.

A Gift
Of Grace:

Occasionally in this book, I refer to Noni's "healing compounds". However, I do not believe that Noni itself heals. Health, and being healed of something, is a gift of Grace. Therapies and supplements, including Noni, simply give the body what it needs to receive these gifts. The applications in this book can help your body obtain all the blessings it can with the help of Noni.

Best wishes on your journey to greater health and well being!

Sincerely,
Isabelle Navarre-Brown
January, 1998

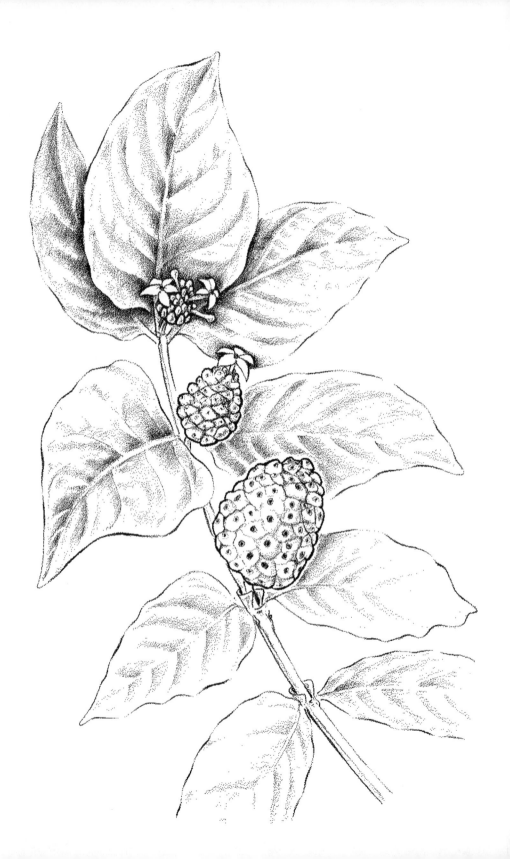

SECTION 1

DRINKING

APPLICATIONS

Unlike juice beverages that we drink by the glassful, Noni fruit juice is taken in relatively small amounts. Most people drink it by the ounce (which equals only two tablespoonfuls). How many ounces of Noni is right for you depends on your health condition, and the way your body uniquely responds to Noni.

We are often asked how long it might take to notice beneficial effects from Noni. Some people notice health improvements almost immediately. A few have to continue taking Noni for months before they enjoy significant results. But most people will notice a difference within a few weeks.

How much time your own body will need to make the changes you want depends on many things. These factors include: how serious your condition is, how long you've had it, what other circumstances, stresses or issues you are also dealing with, and what other therapies and supplements you may also be using. Noni might even enhance the benefits of these other therapies and supplements.

Section 1 offers a variety of techniques for drinking Noni, plus suggestions for acute, chronic, serious and life-threatening health challenges. These are guidelines, which you may modify to suit your individual needs.

If you have several health challenges, select one to focus on first. Choose the procedure for taking Noni that best suits that challenge. Then try the topical and internal Noni applications that are appropriate for your condition. Continue with the applications and procedures you have chosen for at least three months. Your other health problems may also improve as a side-benefit.

If you are relatively healthy, or just have a few minor discomforts (nothing to write home about), a Maintenance Dose may be all that you need. If you are enjoying optimal health, the Top-Dose procedure may help fine-tune your body.

Section 1 has something for everyone, including children, teens and pets. Don't miss the chapter on Interrupting Noni Therapy, on page 19. And please try some of the Noni recipes on pages 73-78. My family tells me they're really good!

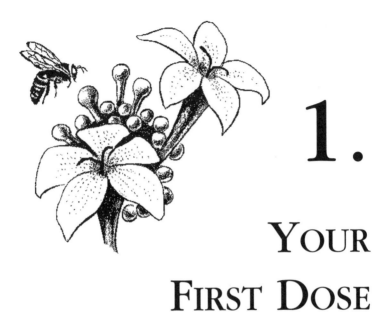

1.

YOUR

FIRST DOSE

Your adventure with Noni begins!

WHY YOU MIGHT
START TO TAKE NONI:

- To improve your overall health and well being.

- To boost your body's immune system.

- To take more responsibility for your health.

- To help your body heal after injury or surgery.

- To help support your body's natural healing processes.

- To better absorb the nutrients from your foods and from other supplements which you may be taking.

(cont.)

3

- To provide your body with certain nutrients that are not found in many foods today. One such nutrient is proxeronine, which is abundant in the Noni fruit.

- To try a natural approach to health and healing, because conventional methods that you have tried have not worked as well as you had expected.

- To strengthen your body's enzymes, cell receptor sites, and other cell proteins in order to help them work better.

- Your health care professional suggested that you try Noni.

- Noni helped a friend, who recommended that you try it too.

- You are a leader among your circle of friends, and often try new things first before recommending them to others.

HOW TO TAKE
A FIRST DOSE:

1. Before you take your First Dose, fill out the Health Evaluation Sheet Part 1 in Appendix A (page 201). This will help you keep track of any changes that may occur after taking Noni. Also read the next chapter on "Evaluating the Immediate Effects of Noni". It can be very helpful to do this procedure when taking your First Dose.

2. Turn the bottle of Noni fruit juice upside-down then right-side up a few times. This will mix the more watery part of the juice with the pulp, which tends to settle to the bottom of the bottle.

3. Open the bottle and pour out the desired amount of juice. Most people start with one ounce.

4. Hold about half the dose in your mouth for about ten seconds before swallowing. Do the same with the remainder of the dose.

EQUIVALENTS HELPFUL TO KNOW
FOR FOLLOWING THE PROCEDURES IN THIS BOOK:

Three Teaspoonfuls = One Tablespoonful
Two Tablespoonfuls = One Ounce

MORE ABOUT
YOUR FIRST DOSE:

After a while, you will develop a style for drinking Noni. Some people measure the exact amount of Noni they want to take. Others pour into a glass an amount that seems "about right". Some just drink a few gulps a day straight from the bottle! However, if you are using Noni to help with a particular condition, try following the guidelines in this book.

To measure your Noni doses, you could use a tablespoon-sized measuring spoon. I use one-ounce plastic medicine cups, which are much more convenient. They are inexpensive, and you can find them in most drug stores. Larger doses can be measured in a glass measuring cup. Use one that lists liquid ounces. When you are measuring a liquid, hold the cup at eye level to ensure an accurate measurement.

Noni fruit juice is usually taken in one-tablespoonful or one-ounce doses. But start with one teaspoonful if you are less than five or six years old, or if you:

- Have a weak stomach.

- Are particularly sensitive to the effects of supplements.

- Are concerned that you might be among the rare few who are allergic to Noni or to the fruit juices that flavor it.

- Are concerned that Noni might cause an uncomfortable cleansing reaction.

(cont.)

- Are taking medications.
- Have heavy metal poisoning.
- Have severe toxicity.

If you have any of the above listed conditions, you may want to try the Procedure for Gradually Introducing Noni to the Body on page 53.

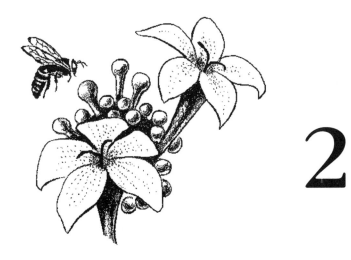

2.

EVALUATING
THE IMMEDIATE
EFFECTS OF NONI

Not everyone can sense Noni's effects right away. But this procedure is worth trying to see if you can. You may be surprised!

USE THIS PROCEDURE TO:
- Gain reassurance that Noni may help you.
- Discover how quickly Noni can begin to affect your body.
- Preview how and where Noni may help you first.
- Find out if your body will react unfavorably to Noni.
- Test your personal level of body awareness and sensitivity.

7

How to Evaluate
The Immediate Effects of Noni:

1. Pour your first dose of Noni fruit juice.

2. Take a deep breath then exhale. This will give you a sense of your lung capacity. Look around the room at objects near and far, to sense the quality of your eyesight. This will give you two reference points with which to compare Noni's effects.

3. Now sip about one-third to one-half of the dose, and hold the sip in your mouth for about ten to twenty seconds. Meanwhile, close your eyes and tune into any sensations you may be feeling in your body. Then swallow. Repeat with the remainder of the juice.

4. Now think about how your body feels. Do you notice anything different?

    • Take another deep breath. Are your lungs able to take in more air, or is it easier to exhale without coughing? Do you feel more enlivened after taking a deep breath? Noni fruit juice is able to improve the body's ability to receive and use oxygen. Are your sinuses more open? Noni fruit juice acts as an anti-inflammatory agent.

    • Look around the room. Do things appear clearer; are colors more vivid? This is a common response, and may be due to Noni's effect on the Pineal gland and neurotransmitter receptors. Noni fruit juice also helps the brain receive and translate information, including that which the eyes perceive.

    • Do you feel more calm and centered? Many people who live stressful lives find that Noni helps them relax.

    • Do you feel more energized? Noni fruit juice improves cellular function throughout the body.

    • Do you feel warmth anywhere in your body? Noni fruit juice may improve your circulation.

- If you have a particular health challenge, do you notice any difference in your symptoms? You may or may not notice changes so soon. Some people take Noni for weeks and sometimes months before they enjoy noticeable benefits.

- Do you feel more integrated throughout your body or a greater sense of connection with your Self? Noni helps the cells access information about their true purpose—information which may have become buried or obscured by disease or free radicals.

MORE ABOUT EVALUATING
THE IMMEDIATE EFFECTS OF NONI:

It will be easier to notice differences in how you feel if you do this procedure with your first dose. If you try this procedure after you have already started taking Noni, the difference between how you feel before and after you take a dose probably won't be as obvious. Here's why. The first time you drink Noni, your health jumps to a higher plateau. Subsequent changes may occur more gradually, or at a deeper level, which make them less obvious.

Also, when your body receives Noni for the first time, it may recognize that the Noni is filling a nutritional need. The immediate effects you may feel could be your body's way of communicating its gratitude: "Yes, this is what I want!"

Changes in lung capacity and eyesight are easy for most people to notice. That is why I used these two references in this procedure. Feel free to customize this procedure by changing or modifying the questions listed above, or the order in which you consider them.

Try using this procedure when you introduce Noni fruit juice to others. Lead them through each step as they take their first drink. This can be a fun way for friends to share Noni with each other.

If you have an immediate, uncomfortable reaction to Noni, it may be due to allergies or to a cleansing reaction. Allergies

9

to Noni are probably very rare. But some people may be allergic to the fruit juices used to flavor the Noni fruit juice. Keep in mind that what may seem to be an allergic reaction may really be a cleansing reaction. (For more information on cleansing reactions and how to tell the difference between a cleansing reaction and an allergic reaction, see pages 209-215).

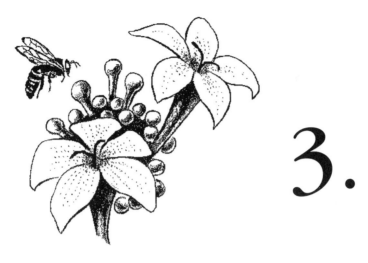

3.

THE NONI
MAINTENANCE
DOSE

Ah, the plain old daily dose...

TAKE A NONI
MAINTENANCE DOSE WHEN:

- You are relatively healthy and don't have any health challenges.
- You know that Noni supplies important nutrients, and just want to take enough to cover your daily needs.

  (cont.)

11

- You are between cycles of more vigorous Noni therapy, such as the Top Dose Procedure (page 15).

- Another Noni therapy has alleviated a particular condition, and it is time to reduce the amount of Noni you are taking.

- You are not trying to test Noni's potential or its effectiveness.

- You have diabetes.

How to Take
A Maintenance Dose:

If your Maintenance Dose is one ounce or less of Noni per day:

> Drink your entire Maintenance Dose upon awakening. Take it at least a few minutes before you eat, smoke, or drink anything else but water.

If your Maintenance Dose is two ounces of Noni per day:

> Drink one ounce upon awakening. Take the other ounce that afternoon or evening, preferably on an empty stomach.

More about
The Maintenance Dose:

The Maintenance Dose may be sipped or swallowed all at once, whichever you prefer.

A Maintenance Dose is meant to supply enough of Noni's healing compounds, such as proxeronine, to meet the body's daily needs. On days of unusual stress, these needs will increase. Double or triple your Maintenance Dose on these occasions.

For the first couple of months that you are on the Maintenance program, consider doubling the suggested Maintenance Dose. This will help correct any deficiencies that you may have in Noni's micronutrients.

HOW MUCH IS A MAINTENANCE DOSE?

- A Maintenance Dose for the average adult is one ounce of Noni fruit juice per day.

- Adults who are overweight may also take one ounce per day. They need not take extra Noni to compensate for their excess weight.

- Adults who have large frames, but who are not overweight, may try two ounces of juice per day as maintenance.

- Adults who weigh less than one hundred pounds may use a Maintenance Dose of one tablespoonful of Noni per day.

- See also "Giving Noni to Children" on page 79.

A morning dose of Noni taken upon awakening may help you overcome the need for a morning cigarette or cup of coffee. Many people can testify, through personal experience, how Noni has helped them overcome addictions.

Taking Noni on an empty stomach can cause discomfort in some people. This is because Noni's cleansing effect often works on the stomach first. This is especially true if the individual has a stomach condition, or any degree of toxicity there. For example, one morning I awoke with an undigested meal still in my stomach. My morning dose of Noni gave me an acid feeling. But this soon passed, and by-the-way, I didn't feel lethargic that day as I usually do after eating such a heavy meal the night before.

If a dose of Noni causes discomfort, for any reason, try drinking about half a glass of purified water immediately before and after you take your Noni. You could also try reducing your dose.

After you have taken the Maintenance Dose for a few months, try Interrupting Noni Therapy (page 19) for a few days. Do this every three or four months. Interrupting Noni Therapy may improve your body's ability to receive Noni's benefits, and will keep Noni working to your best advantage.

The Maintenance Dose is ideal for diabetics because of the ability for only one or two ounces of Noni per day to lower blood sugar levels. Because this can happen in a relatively short period of time, diabetics should pay extra attention to their blood sugar level while taking Noni fruit juice. Those who don't monitor their sugar level and adjust their insulin intake as needed, could experience insulin shock. This is a loss of consciousness that is caused by an overdose of insulin.

Diabetics can modify the Maintenance Dose procedure by taking one tablespoonful of Noni a few minutes before each meal. Assuming a diet of three meals daily, this would amount to one and a half ounces of Noni a day.

Insulin-dependent diabetics should take no more than two ounces of Noni a day for the first few weeks. In the meantime, they should monitor their blood sugar level to find out how Noni affects them. Then, if they want stronger results, they can gradually increase the amount of Noni they take to one ounce per dose (or three ounces of Noni a day).

Children with diabetes can start with one teaspoonful of Noni before each meal. Older children can try two teaspoonfuls.

Many topical and internal Noni applications, described in Sections 2 and 3 of this book, can be helpful to address the various other symptoms common to diabetes.

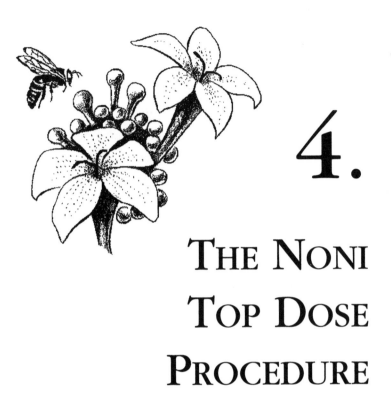

4.

THE NONI
TOP DOSE
PROCEDURE

If you are relatively healthy, here is a way to find out how much Noni your body needs to make significant changes in your health.

WHEN TO TRY THE
TOP DOSE PROCEDURE:

Try the Top Dose Procedure if you have the physical constitution to handle a possibly intense cleansing, and if you are:

- Experiencing systemic toxicity, yeast, or parasites.

  (cont.)

15

- Experiencing a new health challenge, and want to address it before it becomes chronic.
- In top physical condition and want to see if Noni can:
  - Fine-tune your body.
  - Improve your performance.
  - Take you to a new level of health.
  - Increase your strength, stamina and endurance.
  - Build extra muscle or improve the quality of the muscle tissue you already have.
- A health-care professional who wants to evaluate the potential of Noni personally before offering it to patients.

How to Find
Your Top Dose:

Before you begin, fill out the Health Evaluation Sheet Part 1 in Appendix A (page 201). This will help you spot minor health improvements, which may otherwise go unnoticed.

Plan to keep track of how much Noni you take each day by marking the amount on a calendar. Also, each day record how you feel and any changes in your health—even minor ones. This way, you can look back to see how much Noni you were taking when any improvements occurred. It will also help you identify your Top Dose.

1. For three days, take one ounce of Noni each day.

2. For the next three days, take two ounces of Noni a day. Take one ounce upon awakening and the other in the afternoon or evening, preferably on an empty stomach.

3. Every three days, increase your daily dose either by one tablespoonful or one ounce.

4. Stop increasing your dose when:
   - Your physical performance reaches a new plateau.
   - Your general sense of well-being or mental clarity improves significantly.

- A symptom that has been bothering you improves significantly.

This dose is your "Top Dose".

However:

- At the first sign of a cleansing reaction (page 211),
- Or, if you sense that you are taking more Noni than your body can handle,

Go back to the dose you were taking before you last increased it. This dose will be your "Top Dose".

Take this dose even if cleansing symptoms continue. When the cleansing is over, you should notice improvements in your physical, emotional or mental health and well being.

5. Continue to take your Top Dose daily for a couple of weeks. Take it longer if you are very physically active.

6. Then Interrupt Noni Therapy (page 19) for several days.

7. Repeat Steps 1 through 6 when you are ready for another cycle of active health improvement.

MORE ABOUT THE
TOP DOSE PROCEDURE:

The first time you do this procedure, your Top Dose may be as little as two or three ounces a day, or it may be as much as eight or twelve ounces a day. If your Top Dose is large, your body probably has a great need for Noni's healing compounds.

The next time you do this procedure, your Top Dose may be different if your body's needs have changed.

The Top Dose Procedure may be repeated continually. But it is not recommended unless you are physically, mentally and emotionally prepared for change. The Top Dose Procedure challenges the body to a new level of health. This may naturally involve a cleansing on many levels. Please read about cleansing reactions (page 209) before you decide to do this procedure.

Another option is to do the Top Dose Procedure twice a year, for example, in Spring and Autumn. Doing so would support the body's natural cleansing cycles during these seasons.

If you are doing the Top Dose Procedure to evaluate Noni fruit juice, also experiment with other topical and internal Noni applications described in this book. A fair test of any health product, is to take it for at least three months.

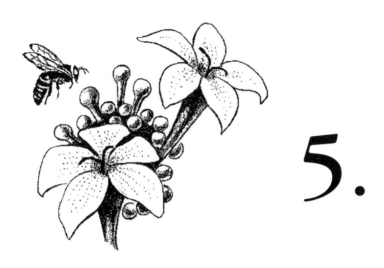

5.

INTERRUPTING
NONI THERAPY

Noni fruit juice can be a life-long friend. But every so often it can be helpful to stop taking Noni for short periods of time. Then, once you start taking Noni again, you may feel better than you did before.

TRY INTERRUPTING
NONI THERAPY WHEN:

- Conditions that Noni fruit juice once alleviated have returned.
- Noni is not helping a condition as much as you think it should.

(cont.)

- Your health has improved to a plateau, and doesn't seem to be getting any better.

- You have been using Noni daily for a while, and now it is time to give your body a rest, to honor the natural cycles of healing.

- You want to avoid becoming accustomed to Noni, so that you don't have to keep increasing your doses to get the same results.

- You want to evaluate how well Noni is working for you, by comparing your condition when taking, and when not taking Noni.

- You want to stimulate the body into a healing mode.

- You want to encourage your cells to use Noni's healing compounds more effectively and efficiently.

- Also, pregnant mothers may consider Interrupting Noni Therapy for one week a month during their second and third trimesters. This would eliminate any possibility, however remote, that their baby might be born desensitized to certain Noni healing compounds.

How to
Interrupt Noni Therapy:

1. Take Noni fruit juice for about two to three months.

2. Then stop taking it for two to seven days.

3. Start taking Noni again. Use the same dosages as before, or try smaller ones.

More about
Interrupting Noni Therapy:

Interrupting Noni Therapy should be done every few months, as long as you use Noni fruit juice.

However, do not Interrupt Noni Therapy if you have immune deficiency conditions, diabetes, or cancer. These conditions require Noni's constant support.

- In the case of immune deficiency conditions, Noni's healing compounds lead the immune system on a course of steady but gradual improvement. Withdrawing this support may cause the immune system to lose too much ground on its progress towards greater health.
- In the case of cancer, pain may return and tumors that have stopped growing may start to grow back.[11]
- With diabetes, Noni's healing compounds may help stabilize blood sugar levels. Withdrawing Noni could cause unnecessary swings in the body's chemistry.

> If you have a serious health challenge and symptoms return while you are Interrupting Noni Therapy, start again on Noni immediately. Also, be sure to inform your physician.

How long should you Interrupt Noni Therapy? In general, those who have health challenges might stop taking Noni for only 2 to 3 days. Those who are generally healthy may abstain from Noni for as long as a week.

When deciding how long to Interrupt Noni Therapy, also base your decision on:

- How serious your health challenges are.
- How well Noni has been helping you so far.
- How you feel when you stop taking Noni.

If Noni doesn't seem to be helping auto-immune conditions (conditions in which the immune system is attacking the body as if it were foreign), Interrupt Noni Therapy for relatively short intervals of one or two days. Try this as often as every two or three weeks.

Another testimony to Noni's truly amazing properties, is its ability to affect the healing cycle. The healing cycle consists of two phases: a rest phase, and a phase where healing changes take place. Both parts of the cycle are essential to make lasting improvements in the body's health.

21

Interrupting Noni Therapy initiates a rest phase in the healing cycle. Reintroducing Noni jump-starts the body into the phase where it makes positive change. Removing Noni from the diet may also prompt the cells to recognize that they cannot rely on a steady supply of Noni healing compounds. When Noni is reintroduced, the cells may better appreciate these healing compounds, and use them more effectively and efficiently.

Interrupting Noni Therapy is discussed further in Appendix D on page 223.

6.

SIPPING NONI

Here is one of several techniques for drinking your Noni doses.

TRY SIPPING FOR:

- Acute* conditions.
- Acute pain (after you have taken a Trauma Dose).
- Chronic** pain, to enhance the effects of the Procedure for Chronic Conditions.
- Conditions in which swallowing is difficult.
- Extreme illness.
- Overcoming cravings for nicotine or other addictive substances.

*Acute conditions are short-lived, start quickly, and are usually severe.
**Chronic conditions last for a long time, or recur frequently.

23

How to Sip
Noni Fruit Juice:

1. Pour your dose of Noni fruit juice into a cup.

2. Take a small quantity of the juice and hold it in your mouth for a few seconds before swallowing. Separate each sip by at least a few seconds, and for as long as a few minutes.

3. Repeat Step 2 until the dose is gone.

More about
Sipping Noni Fruit Juice:

Instead of sipping Noni from a cup, you can sip it through a straw. Straws are especially convenient for taking Noni when you cannot sit up. If you have trouble swallowing, have someone give you the Noni with an eyedropper.

If you want to Sip Noni while at work, bring your Noni in a thermos. This will keep the juice fresh.

For some people, Sipping their Noni alleviates pain more effectively than taking a full dose of juice All at Once, as described in the following chapter. Of course, others find that drinking a dose of Noni All at Once is more helpful. Experiment to see which method works best for you.

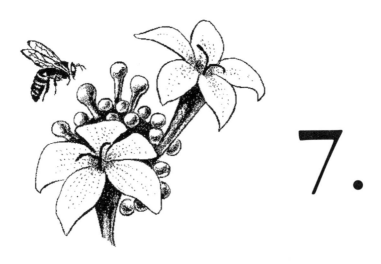

7.

DRINKING NONI
ALL AT ONCE

"Cheers!"

WHEN TO DRINK
NONI ALL AT ONCE:

- For a boost of energy.
- For pain.
- For relatively minor injuries.
- To help wake up in the morning.
- To jump start the body into a phase of positive change in the healing cycle.
- To quickly raise the body's level of health.
- When taking the Trauma Dose.

How to Drink
Noni All at Once:

1. Pour your dose of Noni fruit juice into a cup.

2. Drink the dose in one or two large swallows, without stopping for breath.

More about
Drinking Noni All at Once:

Drinking a dose without stopping for breath isn't as hard as it may sound. Most Noni doses are comprised of only one or two ounces of liquid. Of course, if you are physically unable to drink the Noni All at Once, then just drink it as fast as you can.

If you are taking a relatively large dose of Noni, such as the Trauma Dose (which is about half a cup of Noni), you may have to swallow a few times to drink the entire dose.

When taking Noni fruit juice for pain, try drinking your first dose All at Once, and then Sipping subsequent doses.

Drinking Noni All at Once is most effective if you take the Noni on an empty stomach. The presence of food in the stomach can interfere with the Noni's ability to "shock" the body into the active phase of the healing cycle. This is the phase in which positive changes are made. (For more information about the healing cycle, see page 21.)

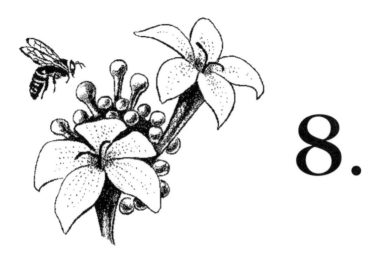

8.

THE AUTO-DILUTION

When Noni fruit juice is held under the tongue, it will mix with a certain amount of saliva. The resulting mixture forms an "Auto-dilution", a custom-made remedy tailored to the body's current needs.

TRY THE AUTO-DILUTION
FOR CONDITIONS SUCH AS:

- Auto-immune diseases.
- Biochemical imbalances.
- Chronic Fatigue Syndrome.
- Depression.
  (cont.)

- Eating disorders.
- Emotional stress.
- Extreme fatigue.
- Grief.
- Low energy and vitality.
- Mental illness.
- Profound sadness.
- Trauma (after taking a Trauma Dose).

How to do
The Auto-dilution:

1. Hold a small sip of Noni fruit juice in your mouth underneath your tongue.

   Make sure the top of your tongue is up against the roof of your mouth. Put the front of your tongue against the back of your lower front teeth. This is a natural position for your tongue, and it will help to seal the Noni underneath your tongue. Saliva will naturally mix with the Noni, and some of this mixture will naturally be swallowed.

2. After a few minutes, swallow all the Noni-saliva mixture. You may do this gradually, or with one swallow.

More about
The Auto-Dilution:

   The Auto-dilution procedure may be used as often as you like. You could even drink all of your Noni doses this way.

   It is easier to hold the Noni in your mouth when your attention is involved with something else. One idea is to do the Auto-dilution while taking a shower.

   After taking the Auto-dilution, you may feel more centered with greater emotional calmness, and have increased energy, vitality and alertness.

   The Auto-dilution may affect your appetite, according to your body's needs. For example, if Noni increases your appetite, you may be deficient in one or more nutrients. The Noni is simply telling your body to eat more in order to obtain these nutrients. Try a full spectrum nutritional supplement, and the food cravings should go away. On the other hand, the Auto-dilution may decrease your appetite if you have been eating too much or if your body is ready to lose some weight.

The Auto-dilution is the best way for someone to take Noni who is debilitated with illness. Use an eyedropper to place a small amount of Noni under the person's tongue.

The Auto-dilution can be used as the Noni equivalent of the homeopathic Rescue Remedy®.

If you have a serious condition located in your head or brain, take extra care to hold your tongue securely against the roof of your mouth. If Noni makes prolonged contact with the roof of your mouth, it can draw toxins from the head through the soft palate. In this case, the Noni should be spit out. See The Oral Detox Procedure, which is described in the next chapter.

If you have amalgam fillings in your teeth that are causing symptoms of mercury poisoning, do not use the Auto-dilution technique. Try the Oral Detox instead.

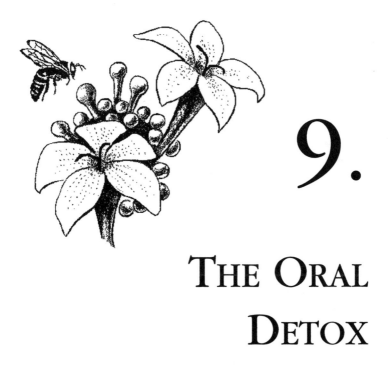

9.

THE ORAL DETOX

When Noni is held in prolonged contact with the roof of the mouth, it is possible to draw toxins out of the head and brain.

TRY THE ORAL DETOX FOR:

Conditions in the mouth, head and brain including:

- Cancer.
- Headaches.
- Mental Illness.
- Mercury poisoning or chemical toxicity.
- Overcoming cravings for nicotine, caffeine and addictive drugs.

How to do
The Oral Detox:

1. Take a small sip of Noni fruit juice.

2. Hold the sip in your mouth on top of your tongue for about 30 to 60 seconds. Trap the Noni against the roof of your mouth by gently pressing the edges of your tongue against the inside of your upper teeth. This will also discourage saliva from mixing with the Noni, although some inevitably will.

3. Then spit out the Noni.

4. Rinse your mouth with purified water.

More about
The Oral Detox:

Avoid swallowing the Noni. If your mouth produces too much saliva to avoid swallowing, or if the Noni drips down your throat, spit some of it out. This will reduce the volume of liquid in your mouth. Next time take a smaller sip. Too much saliva mixed with the Noni will reduce the effectiveness of the Oral Detox procedure.

Even though it is suggested that you hold the Noni against the roof of your mouth for 30 to 60 seconds, spit out the Noni sooner if you feel light-headed or have any other cleansing reaction.

Start by doing the Oral Detox once a day for about a week. Then try it twice a day if you are feeling well and think you can handle a stronger detoxification.

Do not underestimate the cleansing potential of the Oral Detox. If detoxification happens too quickly, you may get a headache or experience other cleansing symptoms. Drink plenty of purified water to help flush the toxins from your body. For other ideas about what to do during cleansing, refer to Appendix B, "Cleansing Reactions", on page 209.

THE DIFFERENCE BETWEEN
THE ORAL DETOX AND THE AUTO-DILUTION

In the Oral Detox, Noni is held on top of the tongue. The purpose of the Oral Detox is to pull toxins out from the head.

In the Auto-dilution, Noni is held underneath the tongue. The purpose of the Auto-dilution is to adapt the vibrational signature of the Noni to match the individual's condition at a given time. Like a homeopathic remedy, the Auto-dilution can then help to normalize the condition, and return harmony to the individual.

If the Oral Detox causes too strong a cleansing reaction, do the Oral Detox less frequently, perhaps only once every other day. Or, continue to do the Oral Detox daily with the following change: Instead of taking a sip of Noni straight from the bottle, use a special mixture of purified water and Noni fruit juice that I call the 1:8 Dilution*. To make this mixture:

1. Pour an ounce of Noni fruit juice into a pint-size jar.

2. Measure eight ounces (one cup) of purified water in a measuring cup.

3. Pour the water into the jar in a steady uninterrupted stream. Meanwhile, swirl the jar for about twenty seconds to mix the liquids together.

4. Take a sip from this mixture to do the Oral Detox.

5. Store the unused Noni-water mixture in the refrigerator.

Wait about half a day after doing the Oral Detox before drinking a dose of Noni. You want to ensure that any cleansing reactions brought on by the Oral Detox have a chance to run their course.

* All fourteen Noni Dilutions are described in my book *Healing Secrets of Noni.*

The Oral Detox may ease head and mouth pain. It may also contribute to increased mental clarity and improved memory. Other beneficial "side-effects" may include relief from conditions such as gingivitis, toothache, mouth infections and sores.

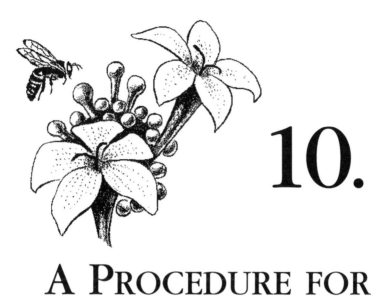

10.

A PROCEDURE FOR ACUTE CONDITIONS

This procedure is designed for acute* conditions that are not serious or life threatening. Or, when you first experience symptoms of what you suspect may become a chronic condition.

TRY THIS PROCEDURE FOR CONDITIONS SUCH AS:

- Bronchitis.
- Sore throat.
- Cold sores.
- Colds and flu (at the onset, as well as during).

- Toothache.
- Ear infection.
- Sinusitis.

*Acute conditions are short-lived, start quickly, and are usually severe.

HOW TO DO THE
PROCEDURE FOR ACUTE CONDITIONS:

1. Take four to six ounces of Noni fruit juice a day, as follows:

   - Sip two ounces of Noni fruit juice over the course of several minutes.

   - Several hours later sip one or two more ounces of Noni.

   - Sip another ounce or two several hours later.

2. Use topical and other internal Noni applications (as listed in Sections 2 and 3 of this book), to address each of your symptoms.

MORE ABOUT THE PROCEDURE
FOR ACUTE CONDITIONS:

Continue to take four to six ounces of Noni a day until your symptoms go away. Afterwards, sip two or three ounces a day for about a week. Then return to a Maintenance Dose (page 11).

It may be more soothing to drink your doses hot. Try Noni Tea on page 69.

If you haven't found relief after three or four days, consult a health care professional if you have not already done so.

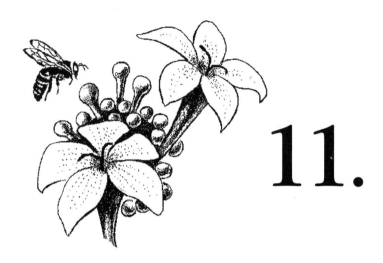

11.

A Procedure For Chronic Conditions

Try this procedure for chronic conditions—those conditions which last for a long time, or recur frequently.

Try this Procedure for Conditions such as:

- Aging.
- Allergies.
- Arthritis.

- Asthma.
- Bronchitis.
  (cont.)

37

- Degenerative diseases.
- Depression.
- Environmental Sensitivity.
- Fibromyalgia.
- Heart conditions.
- High cholesterol.

- Lupus.
- Neuralgia.
- Pain.
- PMS.
- Sinusitis.

How to do the Procedure for Chronic Conditions:

1. For the first three days, take six ounces of Noni a day, preferably on an empty stomach. Take two of these ounces upon awakening, two in the afternoon, and the other two before bed.

2. Thereafter, take three ounces of Noni a day, preferably on an empty stomach. Take one of these ounces upon awakening, one in the afternoon, and the other before bed.

3. After your symptoms improve, Interrupt Noni Therapy for a few days. Then resume the three-ounce-a-day regimen.

If your chronic condition has a localized area, use the appropriate topical or internal Noni application as described in Sections 2 and 3 of this book.

More about the Procedure For Chronic Conditions:

If the third dose, which is taken at bedtime, keeps you awake at night, take it earlier in the evening instead.

The Procedure for Chronic Conditions is designed to promote a slow and gradual improvement in overall health and well being. As a result, the underlying problem can be addressed—not just the symptoms.

Chronic conditions may take a while to improve, simply because you have had the condition for a long time and it may be deeply rooted in your body. As uncomfortable as your symptoms may be, your body has become accustomed to them.

As an added benefit to doing this Procedure, you may find relief from other conditions that you might have, especially discomforts such as: athlete's foot, cold sores, constipation, dandruff, gingivitis, indigestion, PMS, skin conditions and rashes, vaginal discharge and yeast infection.

If your condition goes away completely, reduce your daily dosage to a Maintenance Dose (page 11). If your symptoms come back, return to the three ounces a day routine. After a few weeks, try Interrupting Noni Therapy (page 19).

If you consider your condition serious, debilitating or life-threatening, consider doing the Procedure for Serious Conditions or the Procedure for Life-threatening Illness. These procedures are discussed in the next two chapters.

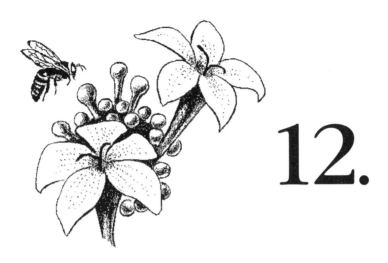

12.

A PROCEDURE FOR SERIOUS CONDITIONS

This procedure is designed for acute or chronic conditions that are considered "serious". Serious conditions disrupt a person's ability to lead a normal lifestyle. Serious conditions may not be immediately life-threatening, but have the potential to become so.

TRY THIS PROCEDURE FOR
CONDITIONS SUCH AS:

- Addictions.

(cont.)

- Athletic injuries.
- Auto-immune diseases and Immune deficiency diseases.
- Cancer.
- Conditions that are very painful or debilitating.
- Plus any illness or disease that is commonly considered "serious".
- Also, a nursing mother whose baby gets sick may use this procedure until her baby gets better. Noni's healing compounds pass through breastmilk to help the baby. Plus a mother may need the extra Noni to support herself through the stressful times of her child's illness.

How to do the
Procedure for Serious Conditions:

1. Drink five to eight ounces of Noni fruit juice each day. Take one ounce upon awakening in the morning, and one before bed. Spread the other doses throughout the day.

2. If your condition has a localized area, refer to Sections 2 and 3 of this book to find topical or internal Noni applications that you can use on that area.

More about the Procedure
For Serious Conditions:

For serious acute conditions, such as kidney or urinary tract infections and other infections, continue to follow this procedure for a week or so after your symptoms go away. Then gradually reduce your daily dose until returning to a Maintenance Dose (page 11).

For serious chronic conditions, you may have to follow this procedure for many months or more, even if you start to feel better. Every six weeks, try Interrupting Noni Therapy, unless it is not appropriate for your condition. (See page 20.)

Drinking this much Noni fruit juice may temporarily cause loose stools. Weigh this inconvenience against your body's present need for relatively large amounts of Noni. The stools will normalize once your body has completed its cleansing cycle and adjusted itself to this volume of Noni.

Sometimes, it can be a subjective decision as to whether your condition is chronic, and you should follow the Procedure for Chronic Conditions, or "serious" and you should follow the Procedure for Serious Conditions. If in doubt, start with the Procedure for Serious Conditions. After a few days, re-evaluate your condition. If you are feeling significantly better, switch to the Procedure for Chronic Conditions. But if your health starts to slip, return immediately to the higher dosage of Noni.

13.

A PROCEDURE FOR LIFE-THREATENING CONDITIONS

Life-threatening conditions are defined as serious illnesses, diseases or injuries that keep people bedridden and unable to, or nearly unable to, care for themselves. Use this procedure in addition to other protocols your doctor might recommend.

USE THIS PROCEDURE FOR:

- Extensive injuries and burns.
- Serious conditions that are not responding to other forms of treatment.

(cont.)

45

- Serious illness or disease that has been getting worse for a long time.
- Times when the doctors say there is nothing else they can do.

HOW TO DO THE PROCEDURE
FOR LIFE-THREATENING CONDITIONS:

1. Drink one ounce of Noni fruit juice every hour. You may stretch the interval to every two hours during sleep time. Do this for three days. You may be taking as much as sixteen to twenty ounces of Noni a day.

2. Ask someone to apply the Noni Tummy Treatment (page 151) on you. This may be especially helpful if you are physically unable to drink this much Noni.

3. After the first three days, drink one ounce of Noni every two hours. (Every three hours during sleep time.) Do this for about five days. You may be drinking as much as twelve ounces a day.

4. Then drink one ounce every three hours. Do this for three to six months. You will be drinking six to eight ounces a day.

5. Thereafter, continue to drink several ounces a day. At this point, try Interrupting Noni Therapy (page 19), for a few days every several weeks.

MORE ABOUT THE PROCEDURE
FOR LIFE-THREATENING CONDITIONS:

This procedure is designed to saturate the body with Noni fruit juice. This is accomplished more effectively if you spread your doses throughout the day. One or more doses may be taken as Noni Tea (page 69).

If you are physically unable to drink an entire ounce each time, reduce the doses to one tablespoonful. If waking up to take the dose is a problem, omit it, but take an extra ounce or two in the morning when you wake up.

If your condition has a localized area, refer to Sections 2 and 3 of this book to find topical or internal Noni applications that you can use there.

If your condition gets worse after you reduce your dosage as suggested in Steps 3, 4 and 5, return immediately to the higher dose. As you start feeling better again, reduce the amount of Noni you are taking more gradually than before.

Noni fruit juice can be taken with medications. However, Noni has been found to enhance their effect, so that less medication may be needed.[12] (If a physician has prescribed a particular dosage of medication for you, adjust this dosage only upon his or her recommendation.) Noni may also reduce the side effects of chemotherapy and radiation.

If you are too weak to drink or sip Noni, have someone give you drops of juice with an eyedropper, as often as every few minutes. If you feel nauseated taking Noni fruit juice, try adding some purified water to the Noni. Or, try taking the Noni in small sips, or with other juices or foods. But keep to the scheduled dose times. Do the Noni Tummy Treatment (page 151), two or three times a day.

This procedure involves a considerable amount of Noni fruit juice. Be sure to have enough on hand so you won't run out. If taking this much Noni makes you feel better, but then your supply runs out, your progress may be seriously set back. Interrupting Noni Therapy (either intentionally or due to lack of Noni) is not suggested for seriously ill people until after they have felt considerably better for several months.

Sometimes, it can be a subjective decision as to whether your condition is "serious", and you should follow the Procedure for Serious Conditions (page 41), or "life-threatening" and you should follow the Procedure for Life-Threatening Conditions (page 45). If in doubt, start with the more intensive procedure. After a few days, reevaluate your condition. Cut back your daily dosage of Noni only if you are feeling significantly better. But if your health starts to slip, return immediately to the higher dosage.

Noni may not be able to help reverse a life-threatening condition. But concerned relatives may take heart in the fact that the Noni can at least help to ease a loved one's suffering.

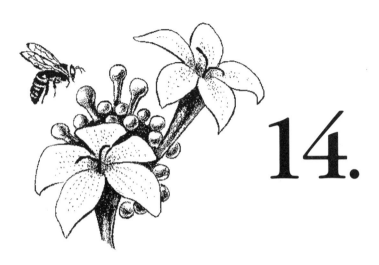

A Technique For Stubborn Conditions

This isn't "heavy artillery", but it may work like it. Varying your daily dose of Noni challenges your cells with change, which can stimulate them towards greater health.

Try this Technique When:

- You've tried everything (including Noni) and a condition stubbornly won't get better.
- Certain symptoms improve, but then return.

(cont.)

49

- It seems you have reached a healing plateau, and can't seem to improve beyond it.

- Your condition is not considered "life-threatening" (see definition on page 45).

How to do the Technique
For Stubborn Conditions:

Use this technique after you have taken at least two ounces of Noni daily for two to three months, and still haven't achieved satisfactory results with a particular condition.

1. Calculate how many ounces of Noni you usually take each week. To do this, multiply the number of ounces of Noni you usually take each day by seven days.

   For example, let's say you usually drink four ounces of Noni a day. Four times seven equals twenty-eight. Hence, you usually take a total of twenty-eight ounces of Noni a week.

   When doing this Technique for Stubborn Conditions, you will continue to take the same number of ounces of Noni per week, but vary the number of ounces that you take each day.

2. Plan ahead how many ounces of Noni you will take each day for the next four weeks. (See the examples on the following pages.) Write on a calendar the number of ounces you plan to take each day.

   Try to vary the doses as much as possible from day to day.

   - Schedule the same dose of Noni for no more than two days in a row.

   - If you usually take at least three ounces of Noni a day (twenty-one ounces per week), you could plan to take six to eight ounces or more of Noni one day a week.

   - Every two or three weeks, you could schedule a day in which you take zero ounces of Noni. This would give you some of the benefits of Interrupting Noni Therapy (page 19.)

3. Check your plan by adding up the number of ounces you've written down for each seven-day period. They should add up to the weekly amount you calculated in Step 1.

4. Every day, refer to your calendar to find out how many ounces of Noni you plan to take that day. Spread the doses throughout the day.

Note: The daily doses given in the following two examples are suggestions only. There are almost limitless scheduling possibilities.

EXAMPLE #1:

Step 1: Let's say you usually take two ounces of Noni a day. Multiply two times seven days per week, and you find that you usually take fourteen ounces of Noni a week.

Step 2: Your proposed weekly schedule could then be:

1 ounce on Monday

4 ounces on Tuesday

2 ounces on Wednesday

1 ounces on Thursday

3 ounce on Friday

1 ounces on Saturday

2 ounces on Sunday

14 ounces total

Step 3: In checking your plan, you find that these daily amounts total fourteen ounces. Good.

Example #2:

Step 1: Let's say you usually take three ounces of Noni a day. Multiply three times seven days per week, and you find that you usually take twenty-one ounces of Noni a week.

Step 2: Your proposed weekly schedule could then be:

3 ounce on Monday

0 ounces on Tuesday

2 ounces on Wednesday

5 ounces on Thursday

1 ounce on Friday

8 ounces on Saturday

2 ounces on Sunday

21 ounces total

Step 3: In checking your plan, you find that these daily amounts total twenty-one ounces. Good.

More about the Technique
For Stubborn Conditions:

Try this technique for a month. If it is helping, continue to take Noni in this way.

The Technique for Stubborn Conditions is based on the principle that our bodies and our cells will become complacent if they aren't challenged or stimulated. Complacent cells gradually become less healthy and vital. Change keeps our bodies alert. Alert cells, by nature, gradually grow healthier. Varying the doses of Noni that you take each day is one way to provide your cells with an environment of change. This can help challenge and stimulate your cells towards greater health.

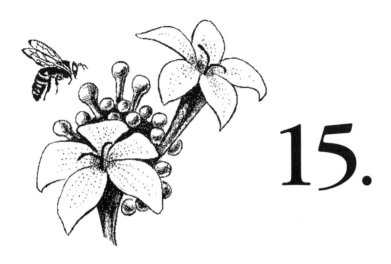

15.

A PROCEDURE FOR GRADUALLY INTRODUCING NONI TO THE BODY

In some cases it is essential to introduce Noni very gradually to the body.

USE THIS PROCEDURE FOR:

- Chemical poisoning.

  (cont.)

53

- Heavy metal poisoning.
- Hypersensitivity to supplements.
- Mercury poisoning.
- Suspicion of allergy to Noni.
- Toxicity in the body.
- Weak or sensitive stomachs.
- Also, if a feeling of nausea occurs when you first try Noni.

HOW TO GRADUALLY
INTRODUCE NONI TO THE BODY:

This procedure begins with a topical Noni application.

1. Apply the Noni Tummy Treatment (page 151), daily for several days. This will help avoid a strong cleansing reaction that may occur if you start with oral doses.

   The bellybutton receives Noni's healing compounds better than skin elsewhere on the body. Hence, the Tummy Treatment is the next best thing to taking Noni orally.

   Proceed to Step 2 after your body can accept these daily treatments without showing signs of a cleansing reaction.

2. Try adding Noni fruit juice to your food for several days. (See pages 73-78 for recipes.) Consume no more than one tablespoonful of Noni in your food per day. You may continue with the daily Noni Tummy Treatments. Proceed to Step 3 after your body can handle Noni in foods without showing signs of a cleansing reaction.

3. When you are ready to try drinking Noni, you may discontinue both the Tummy Treatments and adding Noni to your food. Start with a small amount of 1:8 Dilution*, which is a special mixture of Noni and purified water.

---

* All fourteen Noni Dilutions and their unique effects are detailed in my book *Healing Secrets of Noni*.

To make this mixture:

   a.   Pour an ounce of Noni fruit juice into a jar.

   b.   Measure eight ounces of purified water in a measuring cup.

   c.   Pour the water into the jar in a steady, uninterrupted stream. Meanwhile, swirl the jar for about twenty seconds to mix the liquids together.

4. Measure one ounce of this Noni-water mixture, and pour it into a drinking cup. Seal the jar that contains the remaining mixture, and store it in the refrigerator. Several times a day, take a sip from the one ounce of the Noni-water mixture that is in the drinking cup.

5. Gradually increase the amount of this Noni-water mixture that you take each day. Your goal is to find an amount that allows you to detoxify **and** makes you feel better at the same time. Make more of the Noni-water mixture when your supply runs out.

MORE ABOUT THE PROCEDURE FOR GRADUALLY INTRODUCING NONI TO THE BODY:

If drinking Noni makes you feel nauseated, it may be that your body is toxic (perhaps more than you may have thought). This procedure will help your body become accustomed to Noni, as well as help it to detoxify in a balanced way.

If you know the areas in your body where toxins have pooled, use a Noni Compress (page 89) over those areas.

If you have a buildup of mercury or other heavy metals in your mouth, try the Oral Detox Procedure (page 31) every day. Use a sip from the special Noni-water mixture described above to do the Oral Detox.

Noni Enemas (page 169) or a Noni Colonic Irrigation (page 172) may also be used to help the body become accustomed to Noni. In addition, these procedures will help flush toxins from your body.

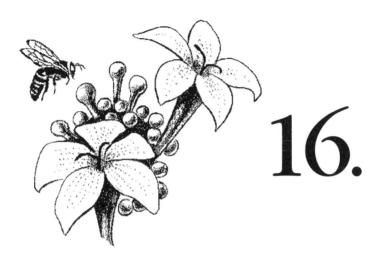

16.

THE NONI
TRAUMA DOSE

Offer a Noni Trauma Dose as soon as possible after First Aid has been applied and you have attended to the individual's immediate needs.

Give Noni orally ONLY if the individual is awake, able to drink and not in shock.[13]

USE THE NONI TRAUMA DOSE FOR:

- Any sudden and traumatic experience.
- Back spasm.
- Broken bones.

    (cont.)

- Easing withdrawal symptoms from drugs, coffee, nicotine, and alcohol.

- Helping the body recover after surgery.

- Injuries and accidents.

- Preparing the body before surgery.

- Severe emotional trauma, such as profound grief, sadness, pain, or anger.

How to Take
A Trauma Dose:

A Trauma Dose consists of three or four ounces of Noni fruit juice taken All at Once. (Four ounces equals one-half cup.)

1. Measure three or four ounces of Noni fruit juice and pour it into a drinking cup. Drink this All at Once, if possible. Drinking a Trauma Dose All at Once is a wake-up call that can send the body into a healing mode. Ideally, it will also counteract some of the effects of the trauma, thus reducing the trauma's negative impact on the body.

2. After giving the Trauma Dose, apply a topical application such as a Noni Compress (page 89), Noni Poultice (page 93) or Noni Tummy Treatment (page 151), as appropriate for the condition.

3. Take a second Trauma Dose about six to ten hours after the first one.

4. Take a third Trauma Dose the next morning. Two or three Trauma Doses may be taken in a twenty-four hour period.

You may also take a tablespoonful of Noni fruit juice every hour or two. These doses may be sipped or taken as an Auto-dilution (page 27). Omit the doses during the sleeping hours, to allow yourself to rest without being disturbed.

Thereafter, take four to six ounces of Noni a day to support recovery. Take these doses one ounce at a time, spread throughout the day. These doses may be Sipped, taken All at

Once or taken as an Auto-dilution. You may also take more Trauma Doses if needed.

MORE ABOUT
THE TRAUMA DOSE:

A Trauma Dose can help reduce pain, and help make you feel more calm, restful and at ease. Tattered emotions may also be soothed. Healing and cell regeneration can be accelerated. Bleeding can be put under control.

If you are very weak and cannot drink the entire Trauma Dose, try to drink as much of it as possible.

When preparing for surgery, there will be a period of time beforehand during which you are asked not to eat or drink anything. Take your Noni Trauma dose just before this time period begins. After surgery, drink the Trauma dose as soon as you are able.

Some people might find it hard to drink so much cold Noni fruit juice All at Once if it is given straight from the refrigerator. You may not have time to warm the first Trauma Dose, but the following doses could be left at room temperature for a few hours.

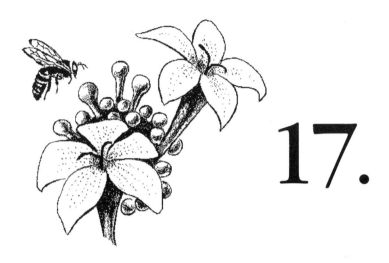

The Noni Fast
Method 1

What? Eat Only Noni?

Use the Noni
Fast Method 1 if You:

- Are relatively healthy and would like to try a fast for general health maintenance.

- Want to experience a greater degree of health, well being and clarity.

- Suspect your body may harbor parasites and would like to use Noni to help get rid of them.

- Would like to use Noni to help clear yeast, infections or viruses.

How to Fast with Noni
Using Method 1:

1. During this fast, replace all the food in your diet and all the liquid that you would normally drink, with a special mixture of Noni and purified water. To make one dose of this mixture; which is also called a 1:8 Dilution:

   a. Pour an ounce of Noni fruit juice into a drinking glass.

   b. Measure eight ounces of purified water in a measuring cup.

   c. Pour the water into the Noni in a steady, uninterrupted stream. Meanwhile, swirl the glass for about twenty seconds to mix the liquids together.

Note: One dose of this mixture equals nine ounces of liquid (one ounce of Noni and eight ounces of purified water).

2. Drink eight to ten (or more) of these Noni-water doses throughout the day. If you feel hungry, sip a dose or two. Continue the fast for seven days.

3. On the eighth day, start breaking the fast by eating foods that are easily digestible. Such foods include fresh fruit and cooked vegetables. Continue to drink the Noni-water doses as before.

4. On the ninth day, drink six to eight doses of the Noni-water mixture. Add a few more foods to your diet. Choose fruits, vegetables, whole grains, and protein sources that work for you. Avoid junk food and over-eating as your body is still recovering from the fast. Add two to four glasses of purified water to your diet.

5. On the tenth day, drink four to six doses of the Noni-water mixture. Broaden your diet slightly more.

6. On the eleventh day, drink two to four doses of the Noni-water mixture. Drink four to six glasses of purified water.

7. On the twelfth day, the fast is over. Congratulations!

   Resume your Noni Maintenance Dose. Be sure to drink at least eight glasses of purified water each day.

MORE ABOUT THE
NONI FAST METHOD 1:

You may fast for up to ten days if you are feeling well and are enjoying the effects of the fast.

The Noni Fast is easier to do if you prepare several doses of the Noni-water mixture ahead of time. As you finish making each dose, pour it into a pitcher. Store the pitcher in the refrigerator.

Fasting helps the body clean out toxins and rebalance all body systems. A Noni Fast does the same and more. Noni has special properties that can enhance the immune system and help the body clear itself of yeast, fungus, parasites, bacteria and viruses. Noni also helps the body's enzymes, cell receptor sites and other protein molecules work more effectively and efficiently. Hence, a Noni Fast does more than clean out toxins; it also helps to repair and rebuild the body.

Refer to Appendix B (page 209) to read about cleansing reactions. During this fast, you may experience cycles of both positive and negative cleansing reactions. The Noni Fast Method 1 can be intense. Consider doing the Noni Fast while you are on vacation from work, so you can get all the extra rest your body may need.

During the fast, consider using Noni Enemas (page 169) or a Noni Colonic Irrigation (page 172). These will help your body flush the toxins, parasites, and intestinal-wall build up that the Noni Fast is helping your body to release. Parasites may be expelled into the toilet.

When you are doing a Noni Fast, omit the daily dose of Noni that you might usually take.

Before you start a fast of any kind, consult a health-care professional who can let you know if fasting is safe for someone in your particular health condition.

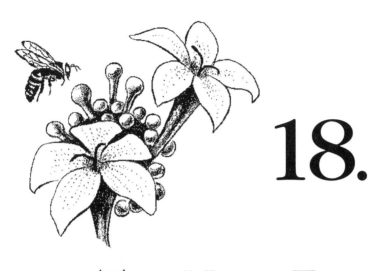

18.

THE NONI FAST
METHOD 2

Here is another version of the Noni Fast.

USE THE NONI
FAST METHOD 2 IF YOU:

- Want the benefits of fasting, but don't want to stop eating or limit your diet in any way.

- Want the benefits of fasting, without having to change your lifestyle.

- Are not interested in initiating a strong cleansing reaction.

- Have health challenges, which don't permit you to stop eating.

How to Fast with Noni
Using Method 2:

1. During this fast, replace all the liquid in your diet (including water, coffee, tea, juice, soda pop, milk products, beer and alcoholic beverages), with a special mixture of Noni and purified water.

   To make one dose of this special mixture; which is also called a 1:12 Dilution:

   a. Pour an ounce of Noni fruit juice into a quart-size jar.

   b. Use a two-cup measuring cup to measure twelve ounces (one-and-a-half cups), of purified water.

   c. Pour the water into the jar of Noni in a steady, uninterrupted stream. Meanwhile, swirl the jar for about twenty seconds to mix the liquids together.

   Note: One dose of this mixture consists of thirteen ounces of liquid (one ounce of Noni and twelve ounces of purified water).

2. Drink six or more doses of this mixture each day. (Six doses is a little over nine-and-a-half cups of liquid.)

   Start with one dose before breakfast. Spread the other doses throughout the day, but take one whenever you are thirsty. These doses need not be taken on an empty stomach.

3. You may continue to eat during this fast. Focus your diet on fresh vegetables and fruits, whole grains, and protein foods that work for you. Avoid refined sugar, white flour, saturated fat, chocolate, food additives and preservatives, and processed foods.

More about the
Noni Fast Method 2:

Try this fast for three days at a time. Fasting any longer may initiate a cleansing reaction. If cleansing reactions do occur during the Fast, drink more of the Noni-water mixture to help your body flush the toxins that have been released. Also give yourself more rest and try deep breathing exercises. A Noni Enema (page 169) might also help.

The Noni Fast is easier to do if you prepare several doses of the Noni-water mixture ahead of time. As you finish making each dose, pour it into a pitcher and store the pitcher in the refrigerator.

People often loose weight while fasting. Since foods are not limited with this fast, however, weight loss may or may not occur. If you would like to lose weight, try sipping a dose of the Noni-water mixture when you feel hungry. This may reduce your appetite.

When you are doing a Noni Fast, omit the daily dose of Noni that you might otherwise be taking.

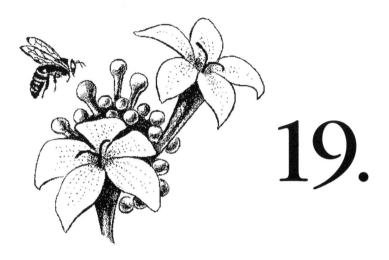

19.

NONI TEA

Adding hot water to Noni will not hurt the healing compounds in the juice. On the contrary, I believe the body absorbs Noni's healing compounds more readily when the Noni is taken this way.

USE NONI TEA:

- At the onset of flu-like symptoms.
- As a tonic before or during flu season.
- As a tonic before or during times of unusual stress.
- For immune deficiency conditions, in place of regular doses of Noni.
- For throat conditions including sore throat, swollen glands, and tonsillitis.
- To help relieve the symptoms of colds and flu.
- To help you relax after a stressful day.

How to Make
Noni Tea:

1. Pour one ounce of Noni fruit juice into a teacup or mug. (Don't use plastic or paper cups.)

2. Boil about a cup of purified water. (Use a glass, enamel or stainless steel pot.)

3. Pour exactly five ounces of the hot water into a glass measuring cup. Hold the cup at eye-level to make sure the measurement is accurate.

4. Pour the five ounces of hot water into the teacup in a steady, uninterrupted stream. Meanwhile, stir the liquids, or swirl the cup, to mix the Noni and water together.

5. Sip, as you would drink tea.

More about
Noni Tea:

One dose of Noni Tea consists of five ounces of hot purified water added to one ounce of Noni fruit juice.

To double the dose, add ten ounces of hot purified water to two ounces of Noni fruit juice. You will need an extra large mug for this. Double doses of Noni Tea are especially helpful at the onset of flu-like symptoms. They may also be used for the Procedure for Acute Conditions, on page 35.

To make Noni Tea, you may use spring water, distilled water, filtered water or pure well water. Do not use chlorinated or fluoridated water. These chemicals may interfere with the body's ability to absorb Noni's healing compounds.

Hot Noni Tea feels wonderfully soothing on a sore throat. But if your Noni Tea cools off, it is still beneficial to drink.

Check the temperature of Noni Tea before giving it to children, to make sure it isn't too hot for them.

For colds and flu, drink Noni Tea three to five times a day. See also Noni Ear Drops (page 163) and Noni Nose Drops (page 183). For bronchial conditions and coughing, try a Noni Poultice (page 93) over the lungs.

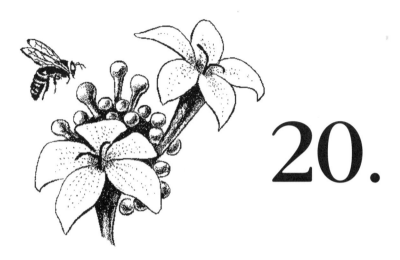

THE NONI TONIC

The Noni Tonic is basically Noni Tea that is taken in place of one's usual Noni doses to help boost the immune system, and help the body handle stressful situations.

TAKE A NONI TONIC BEFORE POTENTIALLY STRESSFUL SITUATIONS SUCH AS:

- Birthdays, holidays, or anytime you plan to eat greater quantities of food, or more sugar, fat, and refined foods than usual.

- Events which may be particularly stressful, such as exams, presentations, speeches, and competitions.

- Surgery.

- The beginning of school (or day care for young children).

- Traveling, especially out of the country.

How to Take
A Noni Tonic:

1. Before the anticipated event, drink a dose of Noni Tea three or four times a day, preferably on an empty stomach. To make Noni Tea, see page 69.

   • Start a few days before one-day events such as birthdays and presentations.

   • Start two weeks before extended events, such as school or traveling, or particularly stressful events such as surgery.

2. If possible, continue to take the Noni Tonic the day of the event; and if the event is extended, for a few days after the event begins. Then return to your usual Noni dosage.

More about
The Noni Tonic:

Teenagers can take the same dosages and amounts as adults. Give older children two doses of Noni Tea daily. Make one dose of Noni tea for young children, and give them half of this dose twice a day.

If your children refuse to drink Noni Tea, try giving them Noni in other ways. See page 80, for a list of creative ways to give Noni to children.

If you are following the Procedure for Acute Conditions or for Chronic Conditions, you may substitute each ounce of Noni that you would usually take, with one dose of Noni Tea. Similarly, if you are following the Procedure for Serious Conditions and would like to take the Noni Tonic to help prepare for surgery, simply replace all of your usual Noni doses with doses of Noni Tea. For example, if you usually drink one ounce of Noni three times a day, instead sip one dose of Noni Tea three times a day. (Remember, one dose of Noni Tea equals five ounces of purified water added to one ounce of Noni fruit juice.)

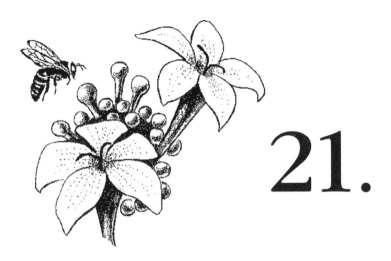

21.

NONI IN FOODS

To obtain the full benefit from Noni's healing compounds, it is best to take Noni on an empty stomach. But sometimes this can be too much to ask of children or other family members who may object to Noni's taste—or even to the idea of taking supplements.

An option is to include Noni in Foods. Eating Noni with foods may destroy some of Noni's healing compounds in the stomach's digestive juices. But other compounds must still work, as Noni is an effective Anti-acid Substitute (page 159) when taken after meals.

INCLUDE NONI IN FOODS WHEN:

- Adding Noni fruit juice to foods may be the only way a child will take Noni orally.

(cont.)

- You feel nauseated when you try to drink Noni.
- You want the benefits of Noni, but don't care for the taste.
- You have a sensitive stomach or a toxicity condition.
- You want to add Noni to your family's meals as a tasty, and healthful ingredient.

Here are some Ideas for Adding Noni fruit juice to Foods:

Sauces and Spreads:

- Mix one ounce of Noni fruit juice with one-quarter to one-half cup of blueberry sauce. Pour this on cheesecake, pancakes or waffles.
- Beat together two to three ounces of Noni fruit juice with a half cup of softened butter. The butter will turn lavender-pink. Store in the refrigerator. Spread on breads and muffins.
- Add one tablespoonful of the pulpier Noni (from the bottom of the Noni bottle) to the jelly jar and mix. Try this for making peanut butter and jelly sandwiches.
- Mix one ounce of Noni fruit juice with one ounce of tahini. Mix in two to four teaspoonfuls of soy sauce to taste. Use as a sauce over vegetables and grains.
- Combine equal parts of Noni fruit juice, peanut butter and maple syrup to cover almost anything.
- Beat eight ounces of softened cream cheese with one ounce of Noni for a lightly colored lavender spread. Add two ounces for a slightly darker color and a softer spread. Use on crackers and sprinkle with dried dill weed.

Soups:

- Add one, two or three teaspoonfuls of Noni fruit juice per serving of canned or homemade soup after cooking.

SALADS AND DRESSINGS:

- Add an ounce or two of Noni to any commercial salad dressing bottle. Shake well before serving.
- Add a teaspoon or more of Noni per serving of fruit salad.
- Mix shredded carrots with raisins, coconut, honey, cinnamon and Noni fruit juice. Add one or two tablespoonfuls of Noni per cup of shredded carrots.
- Try "Tahitian Tuna Salad" using tuna, mayonnaise, chopped carrots and celery, coconut, pineapple, and Noni fruit juice. Add one tablespoonful of Noni per cup of tuna salad.
- Make "Noni Compoti" with canned pear halves that are filled with a teaspoonful of Noni fruit juice then a dollop of cottage cheese. Top with a maraschino cherry.

GRAINS:

- After cooking white rice, add an ounce or two of Noni fruit juice. Use a fork to fluff the rice and mix in the juice. The Noni will give the rice a light purple color.
- Noni fruit juice may also be added to cooked whole grains. Add sesame seeds and raisins to emphasize the fruity flavor.
- Make "Rigatoni Noni" using cooked rigatoni noodles. Add Noni fruit juice to heated tomato sauce. Mix with the noodles. Top with grated Parmesan cheese.

  Adding Noni to tomato sauce is a foolproof way to "hide" Noni's flavor. Try adding a tablespoonful or more per serving—and your family may never know it's there.

VEGETABLES:

- Mash sweet potatoes, then add butter, honey, cinnamon, and a teaspoonful or two of Noni fruit juice per serving.
- Add Noni fruit juice to cooked carrots, green beans and

onions after they've been cooked. Use a teaspoonful or two of Noni per serving.

- Sauté leafy greens and mushrooms. When done cooking, add a teaspoonful of Noni fruit juice per serving.

Meat/fish/poultry/tofu/tempeh marinades and sauces:

Cooking foods that have been marinated in Noni may destroy some of Noni's healing compounds. So use Noni in marinades for flavor, and for its tenderizing effect on meats and poultry.

- Try a marinade made with one ounce of Noni fruit juice, two ounces of orange juice concentrate, two teaspoonfuls of soy sauce (or more to taste), one ounce of berry juice (raspberry, cherry, or blueberry), and two ounces of finely chopped red onion. Garnish the cooked dish with fresh berries in season.

- Try one or two tablespoonfuls of Noni in your favorite marinade recipe.

- Dip cooked shrimp in a mixture of one ounce of horse-radish, one ounce of ketchup, and a tablespoonful of Noni fruit juice. The Noni significantly reduces the sharpness of the horseradish.

- Try a sauce made from two or three cloves of crushed garlic, one ounce of Noni fruit juice and one ounce of soy sauce. Wow!

- Add a tablespoonful of Noni fruit juice per quarter-cup to half-cup of barbecue sauce.

- Sprinkle one tablespoonful of Noni fruit juice over each cup of stuffing, after it has been cooked and removed from the turkey.

DESSERTS:
- Mix equal parts of Noni fruit juice and chocolate or strawberry sauce for an ice cream topping.
- Make homemade ice cream flavored with Noni and other fruits and berries. Or simply use these as a topping for store-bought ice cream or frozen yogurt.
- Add fruit chunks, honey and a teaspoonful or two of Noni fruit juice to plain, unsweetened yogurt. Sprinkle with nuts or wheat germ.
- Add one tablespoonful of Noni to spiced apple cider.
- Sprinkle one to three ounces of Noni fruit juice on top of fruit pies, cobblers and bread pudding after cooking.
- Make butter-cream frosting using butter and confectioner's sugar. Use Noni instead of water or milk. The Noni will color the frosting a pretty lavender-pink.
- Make a fruity Noni gelatin dessert by dissolving one package of unflavored gelatin in two cups of a natural fruit juice. Heat while stirring until the gelatin is dissolved. Pour the hot liquid into serving bowls.

Add chopped bananas, grapes, apples or other favorite fruit. Then add one teaspoonful of Noni fruit juice per serving. Put the gelatin in the refrigerator to set.

If you pour Noni into a light-colored fruit juice and stir, the fruit juice will become a darker color throughout. If you pour the Noni in very gently and don't stir, the Noni pulp will form a pretty "cloud" which settles at the bottom of the bowl.

MORE ABOUT NONI IN FOODS:

The therapeutic effects of Noni added to foods may be less immediate, and not as strong as Noni fruit juice taken by itself on an empty stomach.

The amounts of Noni given in the recipes on the previous

pages are suggestions only. Adjust the amount to suit your taste and preference.

How much Noni you can add to a recipe depends on how well the juice combines with the other ingredients and how important it is to mask the Noni's flavor. Generally, recipes can incorporate a teaspoonful to a tablespoonful of Noni per serving.

Add Noni to foods after they have been cooked. This will preserve the heat sensitive compounds in Noni.

Noni fruit juice has been pasteurized during processing. However, the heating temperature used is carefully regulated so that Noni's healing compounds remain intact. In fact, most of these compounds are unaffected by these temperatures. However, cooking can easily raise the temperature beyond the acceptable limits, thereby hurting the more heat sensitive compounds.

Noni affects various foods in different ways. For example, Noni fruit juice lends an attractive light purple color to some white and light colored foods, such as white rice and potatoes. It can give other foods a brownish tinge. Noni enhances the flavor of some foods, such as garlic, and subdues the flavor of others, such as horseradish. Some foods, like tomato sauce, mask Noni's flavor.

If you aren't accustomed to eating sugar, then Noni might help you handle its effects. Either add the Noni to the dessert recipe, or drink it after eating the sugary food. Of course, this does not give license to diabetics or other sugar-sensitive people to eat foods they should otherwise avoid. But this tip can be helpful at birthdays and other holiday occasions.

When you using a large recipe, you may want to know how much Noni you should add. Multiply the amount of Noni you would like each person to receive by the number of servings in your recipe. This will give you the total amount to add.

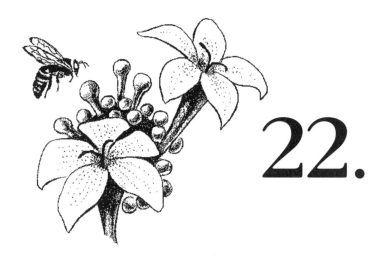

22.

Giving Noni To Children

"You want me to drink, *What?*"

Babies and Young Children:

Healthy babies, toddlers and children up to the age of about eight or nine probably don't need to drink Noni fruit juice every day. They might even resist the juice when you try to give it to them. If they are healthy, trust their body's innate intelligence. But offer them Noni when you drink yours, to accustom them to your routine.

At times, you may want to insist your children take Noni. For example as a tonic to support their immune system before a vacation, before the holidays or before school begins, or after they have eaten something very sweet like a helping of birth-day cake. Some creative ways to make Noni more appealing to children are listed below. (See also The Noni Tonic on page 72.)

Youngsters who become ill or injured will have a specific need for Noni, and tend to take it readily and eagerly. In this case, give them as much Noni fruit juice as they will drink, up to an ounce at a time. Use topical applications freely. One dose may be all they need to alleviate relatively mild conditions.

Seriously ill children can follow the Procedures for Serious Conditions (page 41) or for Life-Threatening Conditions (page 45). Give babies and toddlers one-quarter of each dose suggested for adults. Older children can take one-half of each of the doses. But give more if they are willing and eager to drink it.

HERE ARE TWO SECRETS FOR SUCCESSFULLY GIVING NONI TO CHILDREN:

1. Make it fun.
2. Don't make a fuss over it.

CREATIVE WAYS TO GIVE NONI TO BABIES AND CHILDREN

- Mix Noni with another fruit juice. Or, make Noni Tea using five ounces of apple or grape juice and one ounce of Noni.

- Make homemade frozen juice-pops with Noni fruit juice mixed with other fruit juices.

- Mix Noni with applesauce or other favorite foods.

- Give Noni to infants with an eyedropper, or add it to their bottles.

- Try giving Noni to children while they take a bath. This can be fun, and if any Noni is spilled, their clothes won't get stained.

- Let children drink their Noni with a straw.

- Give children their Noni in a colorful container that is usually not used for drinking, such as a toy stacking-cup.

- Let them choose a very special cup that will be used only for drinking Noni.

- Let them drink straight from the Noni bottle. Though you won't know exactly how much they drink, their body's intelligence will likely inspire them to take as much as they need.

- Play a pretend game with your child. Build a bird's nest with sheets and towels. Pretend your child is a baby bird and you are the father or mother bird. What do baby birds eat? Worms, of course! Pretend you are giving your baby bird a worm, using an eyedropper filled with Noni fruit juice. Worms taste yucky, but baby birds love them. Show your child how baby birds tilt their heads back and open their mouths for their parents to put in food. After a baby bird eats a worm, she ruffles her little wings and opens her mouth for more (ruffling her "wings" may distract your child from the Noni's taste).

- Try appealing to reason. Point out all their symptoms, and explain how Noni might help. Explain that Noni fruit juice can help their bodies fight germs. It can help them be strong and healthy so they can go out and play again sooner.

- Get on your hands and knees and beg. (Just kidding!)

- If a child flat-out refuses to drink Noni fruit juice, you might apply a Noni Tummy Treatment instead. If necessary, this may be done at night while the child is sleeping. It can also be applied each time a baby is diapered.

- Let drinking Noni fruit juice become a natural part of your family's daily routine. Use Noni topical and internal applications often. Let Noni be one of the first things that come to mind when you think about using a home remedy.

Pre-teens and Teens:

When children enter the pre-teen and teen years, they could benefit from a daily dose of Noni fruit juice. It may help ease the many transitions their bodies are making.

If teens aren't forced to drink Noni, they will be more willing to take it. Still, they may watch what Noni does for their parents first before they try it themselves. Let them know the juice is available for them.

Tell them that Noni can be used both orally and topically to help some conditions that are of particular concern to teens. For example, Noni can help clear the skin, stabilize mood swings, ease growing pains, enhance athletic performance and speed recovery time for athletic injuries.

Teens may follow the same procedures and take the same doses as adults. Teens who weigh less than one hundred pounds may take half the suggested amounts.

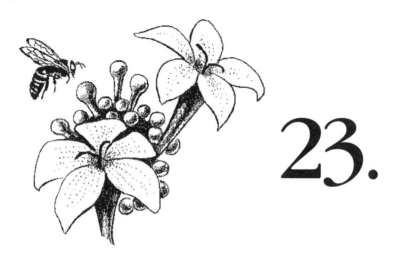

23.

GIVING NONI TO CATS AND DOGS

The following tips for giving Noni fruit juice to cats and dogs are not meant to replace your veterinarian's advice. Use them in addition to the therapies your vet suggests.

HOW TO GIVE
NONI TO CATS:

Some cats don't mind you injecting Noni fruit juice into their mouth. Others won't stand for it. Here is another way to give these felines their Noni.

1. Fill a clean plastic syringe with a dose of Noni fruit juice.

2. Optional: Hold the syringe in a bowl or sink full of hot water to warm the juice. Most cats probably don't care

83

whether or not you warm their Noni. Those who are very ill, might appreciate it.

3. While petting your cat with one hand, hold the syringe with the other hand. Slowly apply the juice to the cat's side, near the base of her tail, or on her hind leg. These areas should be relatively easy for the cat to reach.

   Massage the juice into her fur so it doesn't drip off her body.

4. The cat will lick off the juice, thereby ingesting it.

More about Giving Noni to Cats:

Injecting Noni into a cat's mouth may be necessary if the cat is too old or ill to lick off the juice.

If your cat has long hair, consider brushing her before you apply the Noni. This way, she will be less likely to ingest excessive hair when she washes off the Noni.

You can find plastic syringe tubes in pet stores. They are typically used to hand feed small animals and baby parrots.

Here are some guidelines for how much Noni to give your cat, and how often.

- For injuries, apply the juice directly on the wound. Also give the cat one tablespoonful of Noni two times a day. Apply it to her fur or inject it directly into her mouth.

- For chronic conditions, give your cat one or two teaspoonfuls of Noni, two or three times a day.

- For serious or life-threatening conditions, try giving two teaspoonfuls, four to eight times a day. You may have to apply the juice directly in the cat's mouth with an eyedropper or plastic syringe.

- For trauma, and both before and after surgery, give a one-ounce dose. This will help speed recovery. During recovery, you can also give one teaspoonful every few hours.

- Continue Noni therapy until the condition improves, then reduce or discontinue the dose.

- A single one-ounce dose can sometimes be all that is needed for relatively minor health conditions.

- A feline Maintenance Dose would be about one teaspoonful a day.

Dosages for animals are usually measured in CC's. Your plastic syringe tube may therefore list only CC's. Here are the equivalents:

> One teaspoonful = 5 CC's.
>
> One tablespoonful = 15 CC's.
>
> One ounce = 30 CC's.

HOW TO GIVE
NONI TO DOGS:

Before trying creative ways to give Noni fruit juice to your dog, see if he will drink it by himself. (It doesn't hurt to try.) Offer him some in a bowl either alone or mixed with an amount of water that he will drink at one time. If that doesn't work:

1. Fill a large plastic syringe tube with Noni fruit juice.

2. Have your dog sit.

3. Position yourself beside his right shoulder. Stand or kneel, depending on your dog's size. Hold the syringe in your right hand. Show him the syringe and let him sniff it. Give him lots of pats and praise.

4. Wrap your left arm around your dog and slide your left hand under your pet's chin. Gently lift his chin so he's looking up. He may respond by kissing you.

5. Insert the end of the syringe tube inside the back corner of his lips on the left side of his face. The end of the syringe should be pointing down, between the inside of his left cheek and his teeth. Your left hand should be

underneath his lower jaw, gently keeping his chin pointed towards the ceiling. You don't need to open his mouth or insert the syringe between his teeth.

6. Squeeze the juice between his lips as fast as he will drink it. He will use his tongue to lap it up. The trick is to keep his nose pointing up, and the syringe pointing down. Reassure him by talking to him constantly, and looking kindly in his eyes.

Have patience, and always praise. Sooner or later, you'll be able to give him Noni fruit juice without spilling a drop! (Well, maybe just one or two.)

MORE ABOUT GIVING NONI TO DOGS:

Dogs that weigh over one hundred pounds can receive the same doses, according to the same procedures as adult humans. Give medium-size dogs the same amount as you would give children, and small dogs the same amount as you would give to cats.

You can find large plastic syringe tubes, which can hold up to two ounces of liquid, in pet stores that specialize in parrots. These large syringe tubes are used to hand feed baby macaws.

Try the Noni applications listed in this book that are appropriate for your dog's condition. You may need to modify the procedures to suit him, and some of course, just won't work for pets. (Can you imagine your dog doing the Noni Gargle!)

SECTION 2

TOPICAL APPLICATIONS

Topical applications of Noni fruit juice are surprisingly versatile. They are used not only for skin conditions, but also to help the body heal, repair and detoxify organs and other tissue in localized areas. Noni can do this because of its unusual ability to reach through the skin to areas inside the body that need the Noni's healing compounds.

Applying Noni topically also draws to the treatment area the therapeutic effects of Noni taken orally. This gives you some control as to where you want the Noni to work. For example, while your body may direct your oral doses of Noni to a condition it considers a priority, you may want to focus on another condition instead. So, you would apply topical applications to the area associated with that condition.

Because drinking Noni fruit juice enhances the effects of Topical Applications, it is always a good idea to combine the two. Select a procedure for taking Noni orally from Section 1. Then choose the topical applications in Section 2 that are appropriate for your condition.

Topical Applications are also the answer when people are unable to drink Noni or when, as in the case of some children, they simply don't want to drink it.

This Section begins with a discussion of Noni Compresses and Poultices. These two Topical Applications have the most uses. The applications that follow are listed alphabetically.

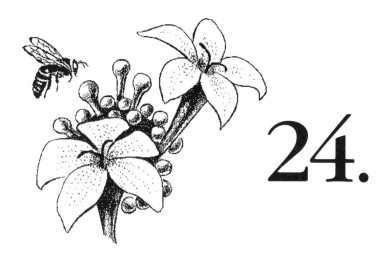

THE NONI COMPRESS

A Noni Compress is placed directly on the skin, to help conditions inside the body. It may be applied at room temperature or with an ice pack.

USE A NONI COMPRESS FOR:

- Athletic injuries.
- Carpal tunnel syndrome.
- Injuries and conditions of the bones and joints.
- Injuries and conditions that require cold therapeutic applications.

  (cont.)

- Painful areas.
- Sprains.
- Swelling and inflammation.
- To accelerate healing in areas where surgery has occurred.
- Tumors.
- Women's labia after child birth.

How to Make and
Apply a Noni Compress:

1. Select a compress pad large enough to cover the treatment area. Do not unfold gauze pads in order to cover a larger area. The pads will need to be several layers thick to hold enough Noni fruit juice. Use two pads side-by-side if necessary.

2. Pour a tablespoonful of Noni fruit juice into a bowl. A tablespoonful is sufficient for most 4" x 4" pads. This is a typical size for a Noni Compress. Refer to the information box on page 92, for amounts of Noni to use with various size pads.

3. Place the pad on the Noni fruit juice, and gently press down on the pad to help it soak up all the liquid. The side that has soaked up the liquid will have a layer of pulp on it.

4. When you remove the pad from the bowl, wipe up any pulp that remains in the bowl using the pulpy side of the pad.

5. Center the wet pad over the treatment area. The pulpy side should be touching the skin. The Compress will feel cold.

6. Cover the Compress with plastic wrap, and then with an old hand-towel. The plastic wrap and the towel will prevent your clothing from being stained by any Noni that may leak out. The plastic also keeps the compress moist. If it completely covers the compress pad, it can help keep the compress from dripping. If you prefer that the plastic wrap not touch your skin, simply fold the plastic so that it covers only the compress pad.

7. If you want to move around while wearing the Compress, secure the Compress to your body. Use whatever material works best for the area of the body that is wearing the Compress. For example, try using gauze bandage, first-aid tape, an ace bandage, a towel or a bandana. Be sure not to tie the Compress on too tightly.

MORE ABOUT
THE NONI COMPRESS:

Keep the Compress in place for a few hours, or overnight. Apply the Compress once or twice a day (or each night before bed), until the condition improves.

If a cold treatment is indicated, such as for sprains, wrap an ice pack in a thin towel and place it over the Compress.

If a skin rash or pimples erupt after using a Noni Compress, toxins are probably being released through the skin. Drink more purified water to help flush the toxins through the kidneys instead.

ABOUT COMPRESS PADS
(AND POULTICE PADS)

- Gauze pads and cheesecloth work well, but so do napkins and paper towels, which are more economical. Fold paper towels in half twice, so they are four layers thick.

- Rolled gauze can also be used. Unroll the gauze, then fold it three or four layers thick, to an appropriate size.

- To cover relatively large areas, use a facecloth.

- Use sterile gauze pads, preferably the non-stick variety, over open wounds.

GUIDELINES FOR HOW MUCH LIQUID TO USE WITH VARIOUS SIZES OF COMPRESS PADS AND POULTICE PADS

One 2" x 2" gauze pad	One-half tablespoonful
One 4" x 4" gauze pad	One tablespoonful
One paper towel folded in quarters	One tablespoonful
One paper napkin	One tablespoonful
Three paper napkins sandwiched together	One ounce
Three paper towels sandwiched together	One-and-a-half ounces
One face cloth	Three ounces

Note: These amount may vary depending on the thickness and absorbency of the material used.

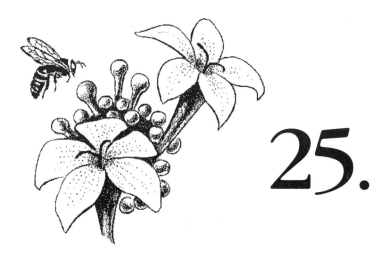

25.

THE NONI POULTICE

Noni Poultices are made with a mixture of Noni fruit juice and purified water that is also called a 1:1 Dilution. The water provides a pathway for Noni's healing compounds to penetrate the body. Noni Poultices may be applied at room temperature or heated.

USE A NONI POULTICE FOR:

- Conditions that involve the internal organs.
- Conditions that require a heated application.
- Asthma, bronchitis, and other lung conditions.
- Diabetes (when placed over the pancreas).

   (cont.)

- Endometriosis.
- Kidney and adrenal problems.
- Liver complaints.
- Mastitis.
- Menstrual cramps.
- Old injuries.
- Painful areas.
- Sluggish or malfunctioning organs.

How to Make and Apply a Noni Poultice:

1. Select a poultice pad large enough to cover the treatment area. (If you are heating the Poultice using Method 1 on page 97, make the pad extra thick to help hold in the heat.)

2. Determine how much liquid you will need for the Poultice. The amount will depend on the size and thickness of the poultice pad you are using. See the information box on page 92 for ideas for how much liquid you may need for various size pads. Remember, half of this amount will be Noni, and half will be purified water.

3. Pour the amount of Noni fruit juice that you will need into a bowl. Measure an equal amount of purified water. Pour the water into the Noni fruit juice in a steady, uninterrupted stream. Meanwhile, swirl the two liquids together, or stir them for about twenty seconds.

4. Place the pad on the Noni fruit juice, and gently press down on the pad to help it soak up all the liquid.

5. When you remove the pad from the bowl, wipe up any pulp that remains in the bowl using the pulpy side of the pad.

6. Center the wet pad over the treatment area. The pulpy side should be touching the skin. (Continued on page 96.)

94

HOW NONI COMPRESSES AND POULTICES ARE DIFFERENT

- Compresses are made of Noni fruit juice alone. Poultices contain equal parts of Noni and purified water.

- Compresses have a greater tendency to draw out toxins. Poultices have a greater tendency to move Noni's healing compounds more deeply into the body.

- Compresses are preferred for joint and bone conditions. Poultices are preferred for organ conditions.

- Compresses may be applied at room temperature or chilled with ice. Poultices may be applied at room temperature or heated.

- Compresses are preferred for smaller treatment areas. Poultices are more economical to apply to larger areas, because the volume of liquid used is partly water.

HOW COMPRESSES AND POULTICES ARE SIMILAR

- Both may be used for pain.

- Both may help accelerate healing, and improve flexibility and circulation in the treatment area.

- Both may soften the skin on which they are placed.

- Both may be placed over areas where the skin has been cut, scraped or bruised, or that has a rash or other skin condition, but neither is meant specifically for skin conditions. For skin treatments, refer to the Topical Splash on page 149, or the Rash Plaster on page 139.

7. Cover the Poultice first with plastic wrap, then with an old hand-towel to protect your clothing from any Noni that may leak.

8. If you want to move around while wearing the Poultice, secure the Poultice to your body. Use whatever material works best for the area of the body that is wearing the Poultice. Try using a gauze bandage, first-aid tape, an ace bandage, a towel or a bandana. Be sure not to tie the Poultice on too tightly.

MORE ABOUT
NONI POULTICES:

Keep the Poultice in place for several hours, or overnight.

Apply the Poultice once or twice a day (or each night before bed), until the condition improves.

Poultices can be applied hot. The heat may help Noni's healing compounds to be absorbed into the body. This chapter describes two methods for heating Noni Poultices.

SHOULD I USE A NONI
COMPRESS OR POULTICE?

If you are not sure which to use, ask yourself:

• Is the target area related to a bone, joint or ligament? If so, use a Compress.

• Is the target area related to a muscle, soft tissue or an internal organ? If so, use a Poultice.

• Would the target area benefit from a cold application? If so, use a Compress.

• Would the area feel better with heat? If so, use a Poultice.

• Is the ailment in the target area characterized by toxicity, swelling or pus? If so, a Compress is preferable.

NONI POULTICE
HEATING METHOD 1

1. Prepare the Noni Poultice following Steps 1, 2 and 3 on page 94.

2. Pour the Noni-water mixture into a small glass or stainless steel pot. Put the pot on the stove over low heat.

3. Constantly stir the liquid, or swirl the pot to keep the liquid moving. Check its temperature often with your finger. Do not let the liquid simmer, boil, or become too hot to touch. If any portion of the juice is brought to too high a temperature, some of Noni's healing compounds will be destroyed.

4. When the Noni-water mixture is hot enough, remove the pot from the burner.

5. Lay the poultice pad on the liquid in the pot. Follow Steps 4 through 8 in the procedure for applying Noni Poultices. However, before you place the Poultice on your body, test its temperature to make sure it won't burn your skin.

6. Place a sheet of plastic wrap over the heated Poultice. Then cover it with a folded towel to help retain the heat.

Note:

- Do not use an aluminum pot.

- Do not use a microwave oven.

- Do not heat Noni fruit juice by itself. If Noni is mixed with water and then heated, its healing compounds are less likely to be destroyed.

Heating Method 2

Use this heating method when you want the heat to last as long as possible.

1. Apply the Poultice to the body following Steps 1 through 7 on page 94-96. The Poultice will feel cold on contact, but it will heat up immediately once a hot towel is applied, as follows.

2. Immerse a towel in a pot of heated water.

3. Wearing rubber gloves for protection, squeeze the hot water out. Fold the towel so it will cover the Poultice.

4. Test the towel's temperature to make sure it won't be too hot for the person receiving it. If it is, let it cool for a few minutes before applying, or put a dry towel between the Poultice and the heated towel.

5. Place the hot towel over the Poultice.

Note: The towel can be reheated and reapplied without removing the Poultice.

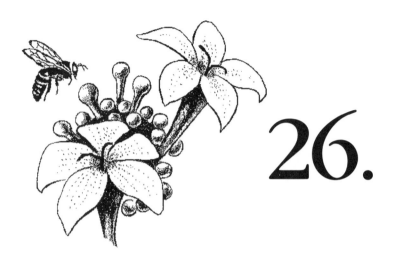

26.

Noni

After-shave

A soothing solution.

Use Noni After-shave:

- As you would regular after-shave: on the face, legs or under-arms.

- For skin which gets irritated or dry from shaving.

How to Make and
Apply Noni After-shave:

1. Pour one ounce of Noni fruit juice into a small container with a lid.

2. Measure three tablespoonfuls (one-and-a-half ounces) of purified water. Add this entire amount of water to the Noni in a steady, uninterrupted stream. Meanwhile, swirl the liquids together for about twenty seconds. This amount of After-shave should be enough for several shaves.

3. After shaving, apply the Noni-water mixture to the skin with a cotton ball or with your hands.

4. Allow the liquid to air dry on your skin. Reapply if your skin is particularly irritated.

More about the Noni After-shave:

Don't shake the Noni fruit juice bottle before pouring Noni for After-shave. The more watery part of the juice, which tends to rise to the top of the bottle, is better for After-shave because it is less pulpy.

Except in hot climates, the Noni After-shave may be left at room temperature for a couple of days. Otherwise, store the Noni After-shave in the refrigerator for your next use.

Noni fruit juice can be sticky if applied directly to the skin. This is why it is suggested to mix it with water. One-and-a-half parts of water to one part of Noni fruit juice is strong enough to be effective, without being sticky. This mixture of Noni and water is also called a 2:3 Dilution.

If you have been nicked by the razor blade and are bleeding, apply extra Noni After-shave to the cut with a tissue or cotton ball and apply pressure. The bleeding should stop faster with Noni.

Noni After-shave also helps to soften and smooth the skin.

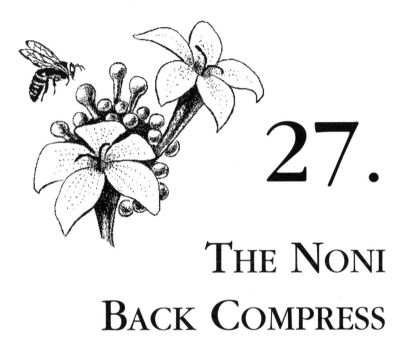

27.

THE NONI BACK COMPRESS

The Noni Back Compress may consist of one compress pad or two separate ones, depending on the application area.

A NONI BACK COMPRESS
MAY BE HELPFUL FOR:

- Broken ribs.
- Low back pain.
- Muscle spasms.
- Pinched nerves.
- Sore hips.
- Sore shoulders.
- Spinal subluxations.

How to Make and Apply
A Noni Back Compress:

1. Have the person who is to receive the Noni Back Compress lie on his or her stomach.

2. If massage does not cause additional discomfort, massage the painful area for a few minutes to increase circulation.

3. Decide what size compress pad you will need and how many.

   - If the pain is over the spine, you will need one compress pad to cover that area.

   - If the pain is elsewhere, say, on the hip, ribs or shoulder, then you will need two separate compress pads.

     - One will cover the painful area.

     - The other will cover the portion of the spine that is closest to the painful area. Back pain is closely related to the spine. Spinal subluxations may be contributing to the pain, and the pain may be contributing to spinal subluxations. The second compress pad, placed over the spine, addresses any connection that the painful area may have with the spine.

4. Make the compress pads. Each will consist of three paper napkins sandwiched together. (You could use another material, but I prefer napkins because they are the perfect size for this purpose.)

5. Pour an ounce of Noni fruit juice into a bowl.

6. Place a compress pad on the Noni fruit juice, and gently press down on the pad to help it soak up the liquid. When you remove the pad from the bowl, wipe up any Noni pulp that remains in the bowl using the pulpy side of the pad.

7. Center the Back Compress over the painful area, with the pulpy side touching the skin.

8. If the Back Compress starts to drip, place a fourth napkin over it to soak up the excess juice. If you need a second compress

pad, add another ounce of Noni to the bowl. Soak another sandwich of three paper napkins in the Noni and center this compress pad over the portion of the spine closest to the painful area.

MORE ABOUT THE
NONI BACK COMPRESS:

To secure the Back Compress to the torso, cover the compress with plastic wrap, and then with an old towel. Wrap an ace bandage or gauze bandage around the torso about three times, covering as much of the compress as possible. The bandage should be just tight enough to hold everything in place. In case the compress leaks, the individual should wear old clothing because Noni will stain.

If the individual to receive the Back Compress is sensitive to plastic, use old towels instead.

Apply the Noni Back Compress at least once a day. Even after the pain goes away, continue daily treatments for a few days, to help avoid relapse. The Back Compress may be worn for several hours, or overnight.

Paper napkins are the perfect size compress pads for Noni Back Compresses. Use sterile gauze pads if the skin to be covered is broken or has a rash.

The naturally cold temperature of Noni Compresses made with refrigerated Noni fruit juice provides an analgesic effect, in addition to the analgesic effect of the Noni itself.

For sudden and painful back conditions, take a Trauma Dose (page 57) in addition to the Noni Back Compress.

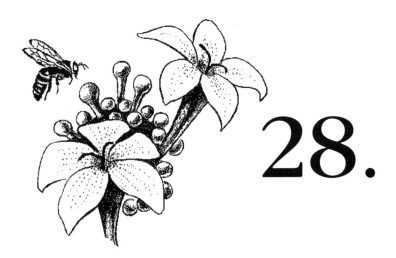

28.

THE NONI
EYE POULTICE

A Noni Eye Poultice can be helpful for a variety of eye conditions as well as vision problems, for it raises the overall health of the eyes.

USE A NONI EYE POULTICE FOR:

- Eyestrain.
- Glaucoma.
- Headaches behind the eyes.
- Infected eyelids.
- Macular degeneration.

   (cont.)

- Pain in the eyes.
- Sties.
- Vision problems.
- Injuries, after first aid has been applied.
- Also, after eye surgery to promote recovery.

How to Make and
Apply a Noni Eye Poultice:

1. Make an Eye Poultice pad using sterile gauze. It should be two inches wide and about six inches long. It should also be four layers thick. You could unroll twenty-four inches of two-inch wide gauze bandage and fold it to fit these measurements. Or you could use a 4" x 4" sterile gauze pad: Unfold the pad once, refold it lengthwise, then cut two inches off one end.

2. Pour one tablespoonful of Noni fruit juice into a bowl. Measure a tablespoonful of purified water, and add this to the Noni. Swirl the liquids together.

3. Press the poultice pad into the Noni-water mixture until it becomes wet. Then lift the pad up. Hold the pad over the bowl, and gently squeeze out the excess liquid. The pad should be wet, but not soaking wet. We don't want the Noni to drip down your face when the Eye Poultice is applied.

4. Lie down, holding the Eye Poultice. Place the center of the pad over the bridge of your nose. The pulpy side of the pad should be next to your skin.

5. Close your eyes. Cover your eyes with the rest of the pad. Gently press the pad over your eyeballs and into the corners of your eyes, to conform the pad to the contours of your face.

6. Rest with the Eye Poultice in place for twenty to thirty minutes, or until the pad dries out. You could also apply the Eye Poultice just before going to sleep at night. If necessary, use a bandana to hold the pad in place.

MORE ABOUT THE
NONI EYE POULTICE:

Some of the Noni-water mixture may seep into your eyes. This can enhance the therapeutic effect of the Noni Eye Poultice. To allow more liquid under your eyelids, gently press the Poultice into the inside corners of your eyes while you roll your eyes in circles.

If some of the Noni-water mixture gets into your eyes it may sting, but it may not. Interestingly, you may feel the sting at some times and not others. Whether Noni will sting or not depends on the person, the type of eye condition, and how the eyes may be feeling on that particular day.

Expect some Noni pulp to remain on your face when you remove the Eye Poultice. This wipes off easily with a wet face-cloth.

The Noni Eye Poultice may help to relieve pain. If you are using it for this purpose, wring out the poultice pad when it gets warm from your body heat. Re-soak the pad in more Noni-water solution, and reapply. The cool temperature of the Noni can enhance the Noni's own analgesic effect.

The Noni Eye Poultice can be very soothing and relaxing. If used regularly, the Eye Poultice may prevent headaches due to eyestrain.

For eye infections, and serious conditions on the lid or the skin near the eye, you can use a Noni Compress (page 89) on the eye. Follow the directions for making a Noni Eye Poultice, but instead use undiluted Noni fruit juice (as you would when making Noni Compresses).

A 2" x 6" poultice pad will fit most adults. Children will need a smaller size. If you are treating only one eye, use a poultice pad that is about 2" x 3" in size.

To enhance the benefit of the Noni Eye Poultice, drink a dose of Noni fruit juice just before the Eye Poultice is applied. Drinking Noni will enhance the beneficial effects of Noni applied topically.

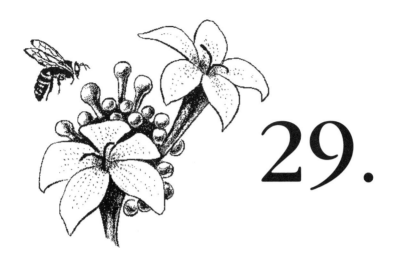

29.

THE NONI FACIAL

Add the Noni Facial to your daily routine to help keep your skin feeling youthful and glowing.

THE NONI FACIAL
CAN BE HELPFUL FOR:

- Acne and Pimples.
- Aging skin.
- Blotchy skin.
- Dry skin.
- Keeping skin looking youthful.
- Reducing stress.
- Relaxing the facial muscles.
- Wrinkled skin.

How to Make and
Apply a Noni Facial:

1. Wash your face using your usual cleansing program.

2. Pour about one tablespoonful of Noni fruit juice in a bowl.

3. Cut up three strips of gauze bandage or cheesecloth. Two should be large enough to cover each side of your face and one should cover your neck. Or you could use several smaller pieces.

4. Gently press one strip of gauze into the Noni fruit juice until it is wet. Lift the wet gauze and hold it over the bowl. Squeeze it gently to remove excess juice.

5. Place the wet gauze on your face, with the pulpy side next to your skin. Repeat with the other pieces of gauze until your entire face is covered. Include your forehead, cheeks, nose, chin and neck. The surface tension of the wet gauze will keep the gauze sticking to your face and neck.

6. Fold a facecloth in half, and soak it in hot tap water.

7. Wring out the excess water from the facecloth. Lay the folded facecloth over the left or right side of your face. Hold it there for a few minutes until the facecloth cools. (This feels absolutely wonderful!)

8. Wring out the facecloth and soak it again in the hot water. Wring out the excess water and lay the folded facecloth over the other side of your face. Repeat this process for your neck. You may apply the heated facecloth to your neck and to each side of your face a second time.

9. Remove the gauze and rinse your face and neck with cold water. Wipe off any Noni pulp that remains on your skin.

10. Apply an astringent to close the pores. Or, apply cold Noni After-shave (page 99) using a cotton ball. Then apply a favorite moisturizing cream.

MORE ABOUT
THE NONI FACIAL:

If someone else is applying the Noni Facial on you, they may use three heated facecloths to cover your entire face and neck at once.

Use facecloths that you don't mind staining with Noni fruit juice.

If your tap water is heavily chlorinated, use heated purified water.

It is okay to cover the eyes with the gauze. (But you probably won't be able to do this if you are giving the Noni Facial to yourself.)

The heat may make your face red and possibly blotchy. This is temporary. If your normal skin color doesn't return as soon as you'd like, do the Noni Facial before bed. Or, try using water that is not as hot.

The gauze strips can be washed and reused for future Noni Facials.

Try the Noni Facial with only one side of your face to discover for yourself the difference just one treatment can make!

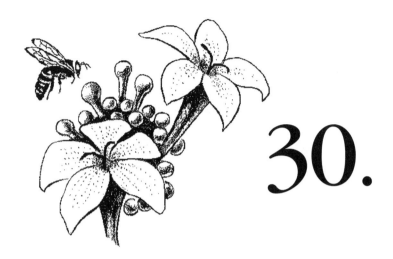

30.

THE NONI
FINGER SOAK

This procedure may be used for one or more fingers.

USE THE NONI
FINGER SOAK FOR:

- Arthritis.
- Fungus.
- Infections.
- Injuries.
- Joint pain.
- Neuralgia.
- Stiffness.

113

How to Make and
Apply the Noni Finger Soak:

1. Find a bowl that is large enough to fit all your fingers. (If you bend your hand slightly at the knuckles, and place your hand in the bowl knuckles first, then the tops of your fingers should rest comfortably on the bottom of the bowl.)

2. Measure a tablespoonful of Noni fruit juice. Hold the finger to be treated over the bowl. Pour the Noni fruit juice over your finger to coat it completely. Treat the entire finger, even if you have pain in only one part of it.

3. Massage the juice into the skin. (If your finger has been injured or if massage is painful, omit this step.)

   With the thumb and forefinger of the other hand, squeeze up and down the affected finger, along its top and bottom, then right and left sides.

   Pick up some of the Noni pulp that has fallen into the bowl, and re-coat the affected finger as you massage.

   Spend a few minutes massaging each finger that you want to treat. (This treatment may feel so soothing, that you will want to massage all your fingers.)

4. Now fill the bowl with hot purified water. The exact amount is not important. The water will naturally mix with the Noni that is already in the bowl. Soak your fingers in the Noni-water liquid (test the temperature first). Continue to massage your fingers, or let them rest in the bowl.

5. After a few minutes, the Noni-water liquid in the bowl will cool off. You may reheat it on the stove for a second Finger Soak. Heat it gently; don't let the Noni-water liquid simmer or boil.

MORE ABOUT
THE NONI FINGER SOAK:

Do not heat the water in a microwave.

Test the hot water before putting a child's fingers into it.

Like other Noni applications, the Finger Soak can help reduce pain, promote healing, and increase flexibility.

The skin on your fingers may become temporarily wrinkled from being in the water. Your skin may also feel dry. If it does, apply a favorite moisturizer.

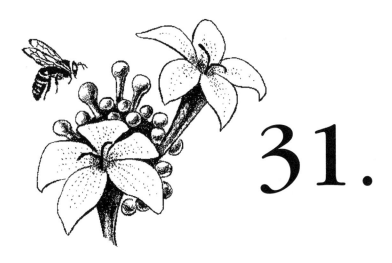

NONI
FIRST AID FOR
MINOR WOUNDS

The information in this chapter is meant to supplement—not replace—the procedures you might read in a First Aid handbook.

> When treating emergency situations—even minor ones—it is essential to use common sense and call upon the help of an Emergency Medical Team if necessary.

NONI CAN BE HELPFUL FOR:

- Abrasions and scrapes.
- Bee stings and insect bites.
- Bleeding.
- Blows and bruises.
- Burns.
- Cuts.

HOW TO USE NONI
FOR BLEEDING WOUNDS:

1. If there is no foreign object in the wound, cover the wound with a clean, absorbent material, and apply pressure.[14]

2. If no bones have been broken in the wounded area, raise the wound above the level of the heart to slow the blood flow.[15]

3. Try to calm the one who has been hurt. Assess how serious the wound is, what other injuries may be present, and if you need to call for help.[16]

4. As soon as possible pour Noni fruit juice over the wound, then continue to apply pressure. Make an impromptu Noni Compress (page 89) by quickly pouring some Noni onto the cloth you are using to apply pressure over the wound. Continue to apply pressure until the bleeding stops.

5. Give a Trauma Dose (page 57) to the injured person as soon as possible. Give Noni orally ONLY if the individual is awake, able to drink, and not in shock.[17]

6. Soak a non-stick gauze pad in Noni fruit juice. Apply the pulpy side of the pad on the wound. Adhere the pad to the body with first aid tape. Replace the gauze pad as soon as it dries.

When you remove the pad, you may find that the Noni pulp has caked onto the wound. It will wash off naturally in the shower, or when the wound has healed enough. Don't pick off the Noni pulp because it is helping the body to form a scab.

Use non-stick gauze pads, because they won't interfere with the scab. A regular gauze pad, when removed, can pull the scab off.

Note: Every time I have used Noni for bleeding wounds, I have been surprised by how quickly Noni has helped stop the bleeding. I have also found that the sooner Noni is applied to a wound, the faster the wound seems to heal, and the sooner pain is alleviated.

HOW TO USE NONI FOR
WOUNDS THAT HAVE STOPPED BLEEDING:

Noni fruit juice can stain wounded flesh a purplish color. The discoloration can remain for a while even after the wound has closed. To avoid this, the following procedure is suggested.

1. Clean the wound with an antiseptic other than Noni and cover it with an adhesive bandage to protect it.

2. Apply a Noni Compress over healthy skin adjacent to the wound. The Compress should be at least one inch wide and at least the same length as the wound. The body will transport Noni's healing compounds across body tissue to the wounded area where they are needed.

HOW TO USE NONI
FOR BLOWS AND BRUISES

1. Cut a piece of gauze large enough to cover the wound.

2. Soak the gauze in Noni. Then place it over the wound with the pulpy side of the gauze next to the skin.

3. Secure the gauze with an adhesive bandage or other material.

4. Apply an ice pack over the wound to help with the pain. Give a Trauma Dose (page 57), if the individual is awake and not in shock.[18]

HOW TO USE NONI
FOR BEE STINGS AND INSECT BITES:

1. Soak a cotton ball in Noni and place it on the sting. If the sting is very painful, give the individual a Trauma Dose (page 57).

2. When the cotton ball gets warm from body heat, and if the sting is still painful, squeeze out the Noni. Soak the cotton in more Noni fruit juice and reapply. Do this as often as you need to for pain.

3. Replace the cotton with a fresh piece soaked in Noni. Place it over the sting. Place a small gauze pad or piece of paper towel over the cotton to soak up any excess liquid. Secure the cotton ball in place with first aid tape.

HOW TO USE NONI
FOR MINOR BURNS:

1. Put the burned area under slow-running cold tap water.[19]

2. Pour refrigerated Noni fruit juice on the burn as soon as possible. (Refrigerated Noni is preferable because it is cold. But Noni at room temperature is better than none at all.)

3. If possible, submerge the burned area in Noni fruit juice. Otherwise, soak a non-fluffy material such as a non-stick gauze pad or handkerchief in Noni and place it over the burn.

   When the material gets warm from body heat, squeeze out and discard the Noni. Soak the material in more Noni and reapply.

4. Soak the material in Noni once more and place it over the burn. Place another gauze pad or piece of a paper towel

over the compress to soak up any excess liquid. Secure the compress and the extra gauze pad in place. Use first aid tape if the burn is small and you can adhere the tape to healthy skin, otherwise use another cloth or gauze bandage.

5. Give the individual a Trauma Dose (page 57). Give Noni orally ONLY if the individual is awake, able to drink, and not in shock.[20]

   • If you need to transport a burn victim to the emergency room, keep the burn covered with a cloth soaked in Noni.

   • Some of the healing compounds in Noni fruit juice have proved to be very effective for helping the body heal quickly from burns, according to Dr. Ralph Heinicke, who has studied these compounds since the early 1970s.[21]

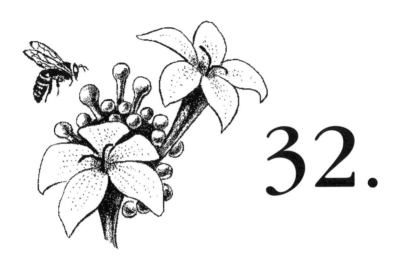

32.

THE NONI FOOT BATH

If you cannot reach your feet, you will need someone to help you perform this procedure.

USE THE NONI FOOT BATH FOR
A VARIETY OF FOOT CONDITIONS INCLUDING:

- Arthritis.
- Athlete's foot.
- Blisters.
- Bone spurs.
- Bunions.
- Calluses.

- Dry skin.
- Gout.
- Poor circulation.
- Sore feet.

How to Apply a
Noni Foot Bath:

First, an overview of this procedure: You will be placing your foot in a plastic bag that contains Noni fruit juice. Then you will be inserting your foot, with the bag around it, in a tub of hot water.

1. Find a plastic bag suitable for this procedure. If your feet are woman's size 10 (men's size 8) or smaller, use a one-gallon plastic recloseable bag. Recloseable bags are preferable to regular plastic bags, because they tend to be stronger. If your feet are too large to fit in a one-gallon bag, you can use a small plastic garbage bag.

   You will need two bags if you are treating both feet.

2. Pour some Noni fruit juice in the plastic bag.

   Here are some guidelines about how much juice you should use in each bag:

   • If you are treating your toes, or the sole of your foot, use one tablespoonful per bag.

   • If you are treating the entire foot, use one ounce per bag.

   • If you are treating your ankles, use two ounces of Noni. (Or, instead of using two ounces of Noni, you could put one ounce of Noni and one ounce of purified water in each bag. This will make the treatment more economical.)

3. Take off your shoes and socks and sit on the edge of the bathtub with your feet in the tub. (Or, sit on the bathroom counter with your feet in the sink—if you're agile enough.) You could also use a portable basin, if you have an assistant to help you. The basin should be large enough so that both feet can lie flat in it.

4. Wash your feet, then put each in a bag with the Noni.

5. Gently massage each foot through the plastic. Besides feeling good on your feet, the massage will helps distribute the Noni evenly around them.

6. Add hot water (as hot as is bearable) to the tub in three stages.

    1. First add about an inch of hot water to the tub. This should cover your toes.

    2. Wait until the bath water cools, then add another inch of water. The water level should now cover your entire foot.

    3. When the bath water cools once again, add a few more inches of hot water to cover your ankle.

    • Cover your entire foot with hot water, even if you are treating only your toes. Your toes will benefit from the increased blood circulation, which the Noni and the hot water help stimulate in your foot and ankle.

    • Periodically, wiggle your toes. Stretch your feet side to side and flex them up and down. You could also massage your feet, through the plastic, while they are under water. This will increase circulation to your feet, which will enhance the Foot Bath's effects.

7. When this bath water cools, remove your feet from the plastic bag. Put your feet in the bath water to rinse off the Noni.

8. Dry your feet and apply a favorite moisturizer.

More about the
Noni Foot Bath:

Perform the Noni Foot Bath daily until your foot condition improves. Skin problems and acute foot conditions will likely improve more quickly than structural and chronic conditions. These conditions may require a daily Noni Foot Bath for several weeks before significant improvement occurs.

Do not use the Noni Foot Bath if heat is contra-indicated for your foot condition.

Step 2 (page 124) lists minimum amounts of Noni to use for the Foot Bath. Feel free to double these amounts for a stronger effect.

As the water level in the tub rises, the water pressure against the plastic bag will compress the bag against your foot. As a result, the Noni will be distributed all around your foot. However, if the plastic bag has a hole in it, the plastic won't cling to your foot as the water level rises. A hole will also enable water to seep into the bag. If only a few ounces of water get in, that's okay. You need not empty out the Noni and start over. But next time, use a stronger bag, or check the bag for leaks before you begin.

To help pass the time it takes to do this treatment, bring a book to read or something else to do while your feet are soaking.

When you are finished with the Noni Foot Bath, throw out the Noni fruit juice that you have used. Do not drink it or apply it elsewhere on your body. The Noni may have absorbed toxins from your foot, and your foot may have absorbed most of the Noni's healing compounds.

After the Noni Foot Bath, your feet will be red from the heat. You may notice that dry skin and calluses rub off more easily after soaking in Noni rather than in plain water. Your feet may also feel more soft and smooth.

The Noni Foot Bath will take longer to do in a bathtub than in the sink or a basin, as the larger volume of water will take longer to cool off.

The water is heated in three stages to help regulate the release of toxins from the foot, and to encourage these released toxins to move out through the bottom of the foot.

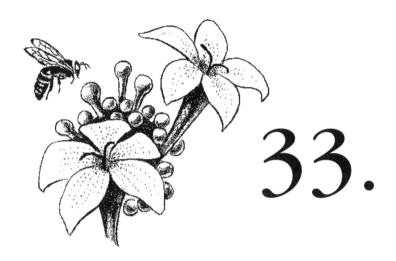

33.

THE NONI
HAND TREATMENT

This treatment is as relaxing, as it is effective.

TRY THE NONI
HAND TREATMENT FOR:
Various conditions of the hand including:

- Arthritis.
- Fibromyalgia.
- Injuries to the hand.
- Neuralgia.
- Skin conditions.
- Sprains.

HOW TO APPLY THE
NONI HAND TREATMENT:

1. Cut a piece of cheesecloth into a rectangle measuring about eight inches by about twenty inches. This size cheesecloth should be large enough to wrap completely around your hand twice. (Before you cut the cheesecloth, check to see if the suggested size fits.)

2. Pour an ounce of Noni fruit juice onto a dinner plate. Spread it around the plate with your finger. You may need more than one ounce of Noni, depending on how thick your cheesecloth is.

3. Fold the cheesecloth in half so that it now looks more like a square. Place the folded cloth on the dinner plate. Press it into the Noni to help it soak up all the juice and pulp.

4. Turn the cloth over. Place your palm on the cloth beside the folded edge. Lift the top layer off the opposite edge and wrap it over your hand. Your hand should now be wrapped once in cheesecloth.

5. Lift your hand off the plate. Wrap the rest of the cheesecloth loosely and comfortably around your hand. Your hand should now be wrapped twice in the Noni-soaked cheesecloth.

6. Insert your wrapped hand into a plastic bag. A small sandwich bag will fit most people. Keep the bag open, to allow air to circulate around your hand. The bag should help keep your hand moist and warm, without being uncomfortable.

MORE ABOUT THE
NONI HAND TREATMENT:

Wear the Noni Hand Treatment for a couple of hours or overnight.

The Noni may get thick and sticky as it dries. It washes

128

off easily under running water after you remove the bag and cheesecloth.

Unless someone helps you apply this treatment to both hands, you will have to treat one hand at a time.

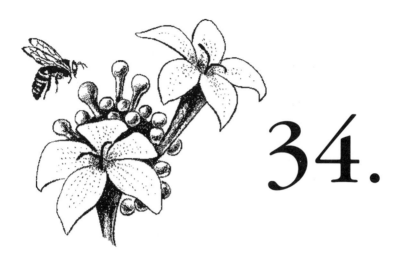

34.

THE NONI
HEADACHE
COMPRESS

Headaches come in all shapes and sizes. It has been my experience that Noni is more helpful for some kinds of headaches than for others.

TRY THIS COMPRESS FOR
HEADACHES THAT ARE:

- In the front of the head.
- Focused in the temples.
- The result of eyestrain.

How to Make and Apply the
Noni Headache Compress:

1. You will need two compress pads for this procedure. The pads should be about two inches wide, and long enough to reach across your forehead, from ear to ear. You can make these pads using gauze bandage, paper towels, or an old T-shirt cut to size.

2. Pour a tablespoonful of Noni fruit juice into a bowl. Press one of the two compress pads into the juice until the pad has soaked up all the liquid. Use the pulpy side of the pad to wipe up any leftover Noni pulp that remains in the bowl.

3. Put the Noni-soaked compress pad back in the bowl, and store in the refrigerator. Cold compresses offer an analgesic effect in addition to that of Noni.

4. Pour a second tablespoonful of Noni into another bowl. Wet the second compress pad as you did the first one in Step 2 above.

5. Put the compress pad back in the bowl and bring it with you to a comfortable place where you can lie down. Put your head on a towel, which will catch any Noni fruit juice that might drip out of the Headache Compress. You may need a blanket, as the cold Compress can make your entire body feel chilled.

6. Center the pad over your forehead and lay the ends of the pad over your temples. The pulpy side of the pad should be next to your skin.

7. When the Headache Compress warms, put it in the refrigerator. Remove the one that you had previously stored there. Repeat Steps 5 and 6.

8. As each Compress gets warm, use the other one. When the Compresses dry out, soak them in more Noni.

MORE ABOUT THE
NONI HEADACHE COMPRESS:

If refrigerated compress pads are uncomfortably cold, keep both compress pads at room temperature. If it is too hard on your headache to make frequent trips to the refrigerator and back, lay the second compress pad over a bowl of ice that is covered with plastic. Keep the extra compress beside you on the bed.

If Noni leaks out of the Compress, try massaging it into your scalp. This may also help your headache.

If you are on the go, or don't have time to do a Headache Compress, try rubbing some Noni fruit juice on your temples, forehead, or sinuses. Wash off any pulp that remains on your skin.

In addition to the Headache Compress, consider taking a Trauma Dose (page 57). Also try the Noni Eye Poultice, to help ease light sensitivity due to the headache. You can do both the Eye Poultice and Headache Compress at the same time.

If your headache stems from a neck spasm, try a Noni Poultice (page 93) over the neck, and cover it with hot towels.

If your headaches are chronic, consider using the Procedure for Chronic Conditions, described on pages 37-39.

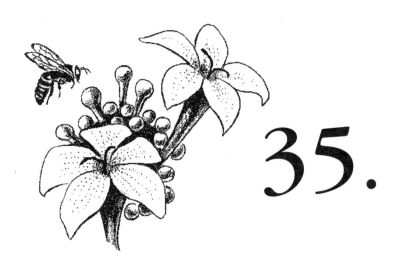

35.

NONI MASSAGE

A Noni massage is a real treat!

TRY A NONI MASSAGE FOR:

- Sore muscles.
- Low vitality.
- Illness.
- Nerve and muscle pain.
- When the body seems to radiate stress.

HOW TO MAKE
NONI MASSAGE OIL:

1. Pour some of your favorite unscented massage oil into a container such as a bowl, cup or plastic oil bottle. (Sesame oil or another lightweight oil is particularly nice.)

2. Approximate how much oil you have. Add no more than an equal amount of Noni fruit juice. Any more than this can make the Noni-oil combination too pulpy and sticky.

3. Mix the oil and juice together with your finger. Or, if you have added the oil and juice to a bottle, shake the bottle. Shaking will produce the best emulsion.

4. Test the consistency, and add more oil or Noni as needed.

5. Apply the Noni Massage Oil as you would any massage oil.

More about
Noni Massage:

The Noni and oil combination separates quickly. Remix it each time before you apply more to the body.

If you plan to use up the mixture within a few days, it need not be refrigerated.

Expect muscle tension and stress to be relieved more quickly when incorporating Noni fruit juice into a massage. Noni Massage Oil can also have a therapeutic effect on skin conditions and makes the skin feel wonderfully soft.

A massage therapist's hands will also appreciate the Noni Massage Oil, not only because of the skin-softening effect, but also because they won't tire as quickly.

Enhance the benefits of Noni Massage by offering the person who will receive the massage, an ounce of Noni to drink before the massage begins. Drinking Noni enhances the beneficial effects of Noni applied topically.

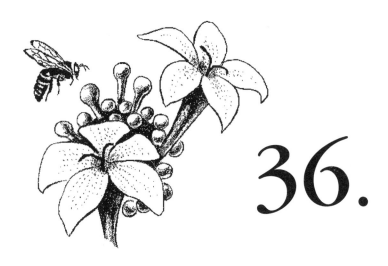

36.

The Noni
Nail Treatment

This procedure may be done on a single nail, all the finger-nails, or the toenails.

Use the Noni
Nail Treatment for:

- Brittle and broken nails.
- Ingrown toenails.
- Nail fungus.
- Nail infections.
- Unhealthy cuticles.
- Unhealthy nails.

How to Apply the
Noni Nail Treatment:

1. Pour one or two teaspoonfuls of Noni into a bowl.

2. Tear a cotton ball into pieces large enough to cover each of the nails you want to treat.

   Optional: massage each nail by squeezing it several times between your thumb and forefinger. This will improve circulation to the nail, and enhance the benefits of the Noni Nail therapy.

3. Dip one side of a cotton piece into the Noni fruit juice. It should be only half wet. The dry part will soak up the excess juice, so it won't drip.

4. Place the Noni side of the cotton on the nail to cover it.

5. Repeat Steps 3 and 4 for the other nails you want to treat.

More about the
Noni Nail Treatment:

Keep the Noni Nail Treatment in place for at least an hour, or overnight if you do the treatment right before bedtime. For general nail care, do the Nail Treatment once every week or two, or every time you cut your nails.

If you have just used nail polish remover, wash your hands well with soap before applying the Nail Treatment.

If a nail problem is serious or painful, do the Noni Nail Treatment daily.

If the Nail Treatment is applied often, your nails should grow stronger and more healthy.

If you do this treatment while you are resting, the surface tension of the wet cotton may be enough to keep the cotton pieces in place. But if you want to move around, secure the cotton to your nail with first-aid paper tape.

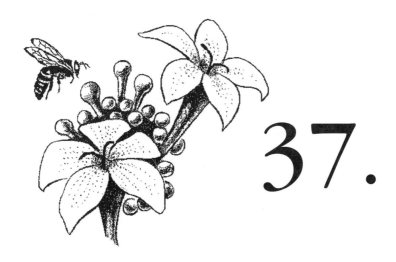

37.

THE NONI
RASH PLASTER

The Noni Rash Plaster is used specifically for skin conditions.

TRY A RASH PLASTER
FOR CONDITIONS INCLUDING:

- Burns.
- Chicken pox.
- Diaper rash.
- Eczema.
- Hives.
- Liver spots.
- Pimples and acne.

- Poison Ivy.
- Psoriasis.
- Scars.
- Skin eruptions.
- Stretch marks.

How to Make and Apply
A Noni Rash Plaster:

1. Select a plaster pad that will cover the area you want to treat. You may use cheesecloth, an unfolded sterile gauze pad, a piece of an old T-shirt or a paper towel. A plaster pad is thinner than a compress pad or poultice pad.

2. Pour some Noni fruit juice into a bowl. The amount of Noni you will need depends on the size of the plaster cloth you are using. Start with one-half tablespoonful of Noni, and add more if needed.

   If your plaster pad is bigger than four inches square, pour the Noni onto a dinner plate. This will make it easier to distribute the Noni evenly throughout the plaster pad.

3. Press the plaster cloth into the juice. Do not turn the cloth over.

4. Hold the cloth over the bowl and squeeze the cloth gently so excess juice can drip off. The cloth should be wet, but not dripping wet.

5. Lay the Noni Rash Plaster over the treatment area to cover it. The pulpy side of the cloth should be touching the skin. The plaster will feel cold at first, but body heat will soon warm it.

6. Press the Rash Plaster onto the skin and mold it around the contours of your body. The Plaster will be slightly adhesive; perhaps just enough that you won't need to secure it in place. If you do need to secure it, don't use plastic. In this case, you want the area to breathe—the skin heals better that way. Try wrapping the plaster pad with gauze bandage instead.

   Apply additional plaster pads as needed to completely cover all the skin to be treated. The Rash Plaster can cover a considerably large portion of the body if necessary.

7. Leave the Rash Plaster in place until it dries. Then rinse out the cloth, soak it in more Noni, and reapply.

MORE ABOUT THE
NONI RASH PLASTER:

Apply the Rash Plaster as often as needed.

In cases of contagious rashes, such as Poison Ivy, you may leave the Rash Plaster in place even when it dries out. This may prevent the rash from spreading. But keeping the plaster wet with Noni may help control the itching.

Think twice before using the Noni Rash Plaster for pimples or acne on the face. Noni fruit juice will stain open skin a purple color.

For diaper rash, apply the Noni Rash Plaster on the reddened area. Then put on the diaper. The diaper will hold the Plaster in place. When you change the diaper, throw out the plaster pad. Then reapply the Rash Plaster using a clean plaster pad soaked in more Noni. My baby's diaper rashes have cleared up remarkably quickly using this technique.

To warm the Rash Plaster before placing it on your baby's bottom, prepare the Plaster as in Steps 1 through 3, but use a glass bowl. Add a few inches of very hot tap water to the bathroom sink. Place the bowl, which contains the Noni-soaked Rash Plaster, in the hot water to warm. Be sure none of the water gets into the bowl. In the meantime, clean up the baby. By the time you are ready to apply the Rash Plaster, it should be warm. Test its temperature before you place it on the baby.

38.

THE NONI
SCALP TREATMENT

This treatment won't turn your hair purple!

TRY THE NONI
SCALP TREATMENT FOR:

Various scalp conditions including:

- Dandruff.
- Eczema.
- Psoriasis.
- Itchy scalp.
- Scalp sores.

143

How to Apply the
Noni Scalp Treatment:

1. Pour some Noni fruit juice in a medicine cup or small plastic cup. You will need at least one tablespoonful. Use as much as two ounces if your condition is throughout your scalp, if you have a lot of hair, or if your condition is relatively severe.

2. Wrap a towel around your neck and shoulders.

3. Hold the cup with the Noni over your head. Part the hair over a section of your scalp. Pour some of the juice on this area so the Noni makes direct contact with your skin. As you pour the juice on, massage it into your hair so it does not drip off your head.

4. Repeat Step 3 with different sections of your scalp. Apply the Noni to your entire scalp, or just those areas that need it. Put a second and third coat of juice over problem areas.

5. When you have applied all the Noni, massage it into your scalp for a few minutes.

6. Brush or comb your hair. Then let it air dry, or cover your head with a towel or an old shower-cap.

7. Keep the Noni on for a few hours, or overnight, or just until it dries. Then rinse out the Noni fruit juice and wash your hair.

More about the
Noni Scalp Treatment:

Repeat this procedure daily until the condition improves.

You may need someone's help to do this procedure, especially if you find it difficult to reach your arms up over your head.

If you have little or no hair, the Noni Rash Plaster (page 139), may work better for you.

Besides having a therapeutic effect on scalp conditions, the Noni Scalp Treatment may also help to alleviate headaches.

If you do this treatment before bed, cover your pillowcase with a towel to prevent the juice from staining it.

Noni fruit juice applied to your scalp acts somewhat like styling gel—with a fruity fragrance.

In researching whether Noni can be used safely on the hair, I collected many hair samples that included natural, treated, as well as gray hair. Part of each sample was soaked in Noni fruit juice for over twenty-four hours, and then studied. I also examined the samples under a microscope.

Noni appeared to have no negative effect on the natural and gray hair samples. I noticed that after using Noni on my own scalp (I kept it there until it dried, and then washed it off), my natural hair seemed softer and to have more "body".

The effects of Noni on treated hair varied. This is not surprising, since there are so many different kinds of hair treatments. My conclusion was this: just to be safe, those who have treated hair and wish to do the Noni Scalp Treatment, should wash off the Noni after about twenty to thirty minutes. This amount of time will allow the Noni to work on your scalp, while not interfering with your hair treatment.

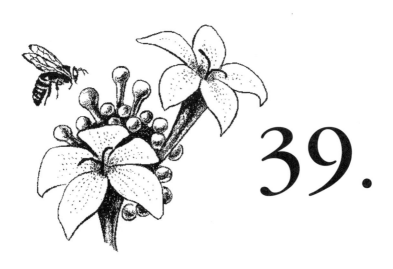

THE NONI SMALL AREA TREATMENT

This is also called a "Mini Compress."

USE THE NONI SMALL AREA TREATMENT FOR:

- Bee stings.
- Boils and abscesses.
- Infected pierced earring holes.
- Insect and spider bites.
- Moles.
- Puncture wounds.
- Single pimples or acne.

- Small bruises.
- Small scars.
- Warts.

147

How to Make and Apply
The Noni Small Area Treatment:

1. Tear off a one-half inch piece of a cotton ball. Shape this cotton piece so it is somewhat round.

   If the target area is a relatively large abscess, bruise or scar, you may need to use a whole cotton ball. Also use a whole cotton ball if the target area is painful.

2. Dip the cotton in Noni fruit juice, so half of it is wet.

3. Place the wet side of the cotton over the target area.

4. The surface tension of the wet cotton may be enough to keep the cotton attached to your skin, even if you move around. If the target area is underneath clothing, or if you are particularly active, you may secure the cotton with first-aid tape or with an adhesive bandage.

More about the Noni
Small Area Treatment:

Most conditions for which this Mini-compress is applied clear up more quickly if you use the pulpier part of the Noni fruit juice. So be sure to gently shake the Noni bottle before pouring Noni to treat small areas.

Wet only half the cotton ball so that the dry portion can soak up excess liquid. This will prevent the Mini-compress from leaking.

Some moles, warts and small scars may require daily application for a few weeks before you notice significant changes. Try applying the Noni Small Area Treatment on these areas every night before bed. Acute problems may require only a few applications.

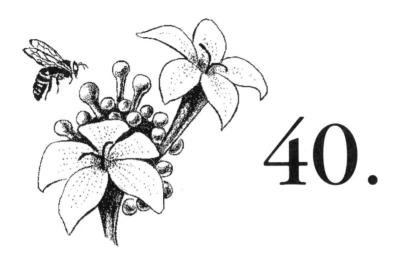

40.

THE NONI
TOPICAL SPLASH

The Topical Splash is helpful for skin conditions that cover relatively large areas, or when you need quick relief when on the go.

USE A NONI TOPICAL SPLASH FOR:

- Allergic reactions.
- Burns.
- Chicken pox.
- Eczema.
- Pimples and acne.
- Poison ivy.
- Psoriasis.
- Rashes.
- Skin irritations.
- Sunburn.

149

HOW TO APPLY A
NONI TOPICAL SPLASH:

1. Pour an ounce of Noni fruit juice in a small glass bottle or container.

2. Measure three tablespoonfuls (one-and-a-half ounces) of purified water. Pour the water into the Noni in a steady, uninterrupted stream. Meanwhile, swirl the bottle for about twenty seconds to mix the liquids together.

3. Apply the Noni-water mixture to the skin with a cotton ball, or splash it on with the palm of your hand. If the glass bottle you use has an eyedropper for a lid, then applying the Topical Splash is even easier. Use the eyedropper to place a few drops of the Noni-water mixture on your skin. Then gently rub the Noni around the area with your hand.

4. When the liquid dries (usually no more than a minute), apply the Noni a second time and possibly a third time.

5. Use the Topical Splash as often during the day as you like. Repeat the Splash daily as needed.

MORE ABOUT THE
NONI TOPICAL SPLASH:

Don't shake the Noni bottle before pouring. Skin conditions respond better to the watery part of the Noni fruit juice, which tends to rise to the top of the Noni bottle. Using the pulpy part can leave pulp remnants on the skin.

Noni by itself can feel sticky when applied to the skin. Adding one-and-a-half parts of purified water dilutes the Noni just enough to keep it effective, without becoming sticky. This ratio of Noni and water will not give the skin a purple cast.

The Topical Splash can leave the skin feeling soft and smooth. It can also reduce itchiness and irritation on contact.

Store the Topical Splash in a small glass jar or tincture bottle. Keep it in the refrigerator when you are not carrying it with you.

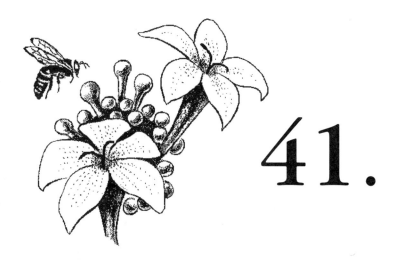

THE NONI TUMMY TREATMENT

The Noni Tummy Treatment is used on the lower abdomen, over and below the bellybutton.

USE THE NONI
TUMMY TREATMENT WHEN:

- A child is ill.
- A child refuses to drink Noni.
- An individual is in a coma or has lost consciousness and you and a medical team have done everything else you can do.
- Drinking Noni causes nausea.

  (cont.)

151

- Drinking Noni causes a too strong cleansing reaction.
- You are unable to take liquids orally.
- You want to benefit from Noni, but are allergic to it or are hypersensitive to its effects.
- You want to support the body through a fever.

The Noni Tummy
Treatment is also Helpful for:

- Conditions of the intestine and abdomen.
- Endometriosis.
- Heavy metal or chemical toxicity.
- Systemic candida.
- Intestinal parasite infestation.

How to Apply a
Noni Tummy Treatment:

1. Select a compress pad:

   - Use a 2" x 2" gauze pad for infants and a 4" x 4" gauze pad for babies.

   - For children, teens, and adults with somewhat flat tummies, use a paper napkin for the compress pad. Paper napkins are about six inches square, and large enough to cover the required area.

   - Adults with larger tummies can use a compress pad made of a facecloth, or three paper towels laid one on top of the other, like a sandwich.

2. Heat a glass bowl by pouring very hot tap water or heated water into it. After several seconds, when the bowl is hot, pour out the water and quickly dry the bowl.

3. Pour the amount of Noni fruit juice that you will need into the heated bowl. (See the information box on page 92 for an idea of how much liquid you may need.)

4. Place the compress pad on the Noni fruit juice, and gently press down on the pad to help it soak up all the liquid. When you remove the pad from the bowl, wipe up any pulp that remains in the bowl with the pulpy side of the pad.

5. Place the wet pad over the lower abdomen, such that the top one inch of the pad completely covers the bellybutton. People who are overweight should center the Tummy Treatment over the bellybutton. The pulpy side of the pad should be touching the skin.

6. Cover the compress pad with plastic wrap, and then with an old hand-towel.

MORE ABOUT THE
NONI TUMMY TREATMENT:

A Noni Tummy Treatment may be made with Noni alone, or with equal parts of Noni and purified water.

- It is easier, and preferable to use undiluted Noni when applying the Tummy Treatment on babies and children.

- Adults who are using a facecloth or paper towels for a compress pad may need two or three ounces or more of Noni. If they would prefer a more economical application, they may dilute the Noni with an equal amount of purified water. Diluting the Noni with this proportion of water may actually help the Noni healing compounds reach into the adult body.

If you are adding water:

1. Measure the amount of Noni you will need and pour it into the heated bowl.

2. Measure an equal amount of purified water and add this to the Noni in a slow, steady stream.

3. Swirl the two liquids together, or stir them briefly with your finger. Then wet the poultice pad.

Keep the Tummy Treatment in place for at least a few hours. Apply it once or twice a day, or as often as needed until the condition improves.

People who prefer to sleep on their back could apply the Tummy Treatment at night, just before going to bed.

If the compress pad cools off by the time you are ready to apply it to the body, leave the pad in the bowl of Noni. Then place the bottom half of the bowl in a container or sink full of hot water. Apply the compress pad when it is warmed enough for you.

For babies who are ill, give the Tummy Treatment each time you do a diaper change. A gauze pad can completely cover their lower tummies. The diaper will hold the Tummy Treatment in place, so you won't need plastic wrap for that purpose. Besides, the plastic might irritate their delicate skin. However, you may use a piece of plastic folded to the same size as the compress pad to cover the Tummy Treatment. This will prevent the diaper from soaking up the Noni. The diaper will protect the clothing from being stained, but you may need a larger sized diaper than usual.

Adults could hold the Tummy Treatment in place by wearing it inside a pair of pants. Select a pair that you don't mind getting stained, in case some Noni fruit juice leaks out. This method allows you to move around, without anyone knowing that you are wearing a compress pad.

There are two ways to place the compress pad on the body.

1. Have the upper edge parallel to the body's midline. This edge should overlap the bellybutton by about an inch.

2. Place the pad diagonally on the body, with the upper corner of the pad covering the bellybutton.

Tummy Treatments are the next best thing to drinking Noni for two reasons. First, Noni's healing compounds enter the body through the bellybutton more quickly than through skin elsewhere on the body (except under the tongue). Second, the Noni healing compounds that enter the body through the bellybutton tend to remain in the abdominal area and work there, rather than spreading throughout the body as they do when taken orally.

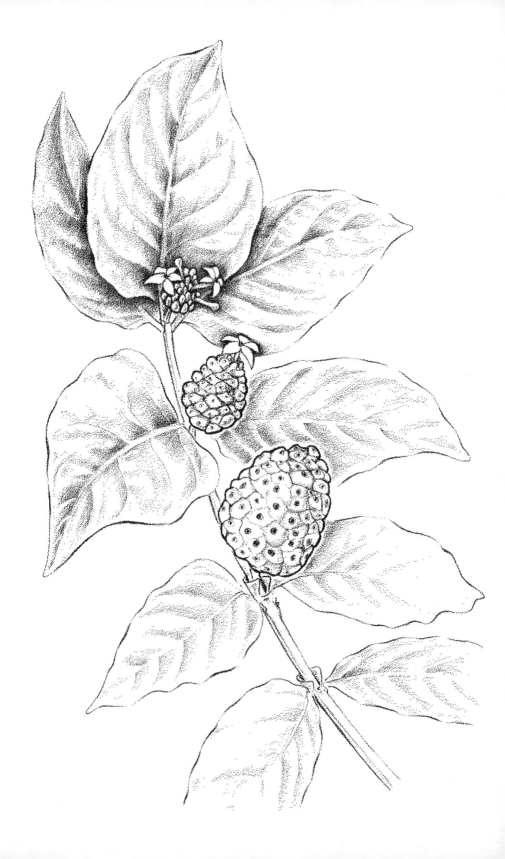

SECTION 3

OTHER INTERNAL APPLICATIONS OF NONI

Drinking Noni and applying it topically are the two most obvious uses of Noni. But this remarkable juice can also be therapeutic in ways that one might not expect. If it seems too odd to try putting fruit juice in your nose or ears, for example, don't think of Noni as a juice drink. Think of it as the liquid extract of an amazing tropical fruit, which contains special healing compounds.

This Section describes procedures for many internal applications of Noni fruit juice. The applications are listed alphabetically.

When you use internal applications, plan to drink Noni as well. Oral and internal Noni applications will enhance each other's benefits. To decide how much Noni fruit juice to take orally, select a procedure in Section 1 that best suits your condition. Internal applications also draw the the healing compounds from the Noni that you drink to those parts of the body where the Noni is applied.

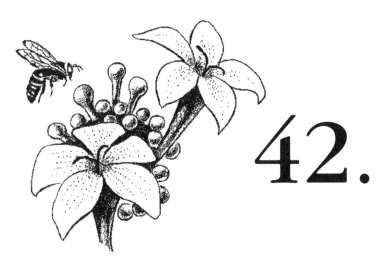

THE NONI
ANTI-ACID
SUBSTITUTE

Though Noni does not work in the same way as regular anti-acids, the end results are often just as relieving.

TRY THE NONI
ANTI-ACID SUBSTITUTE FOR:

• Heartburn.

• Indigestion.

• Stomach distress from overeating.
  (cont.)

159

- Also, if you are relatively healthy, but unaccustomed to certain foods like refined sugar, meat or "junk" food, Noni may help your body handle these foods on those special occasions when you do eat them.

How to use Noni
As an Anti-acid Substitute:

1. Drink one ounce of Noni following your meal, either before or after symptoms arise.

2. If you don't feel better after a few minutes, try drinking another ounce.

More about the
Noni Anti-acid Substitute:

The Noni-Anti-acid Substitute, whereby you take Noni after a meal, will address the symptoms of a stomach condition. Whereas taking Noni on an empty stomach will help treat the underlying cause of the stomach distress.

Try the Procedure for Chronic Conditions (page 37), which suggests taking three ounces of Noni a day. Take one of these three ounces a few minutes before each meal. Then eat mindfully. If you still feel distress afterwards, take a tablespoonful or more of Noni after the meal. Eventually, you may not need the Noni Anti-acid Substitute any more.

Taking an ounce of Noni before each meal can also help curb your appetite if you tend to overeat.

The Noni Fast Method 2 (page 65) is another approach to dealing with chronic indigestion and heartburn. If you do the Fast to help a stomach condition, take some of the Noni-water mixture (page 66) that is used for the Fast, both before and after each meal.

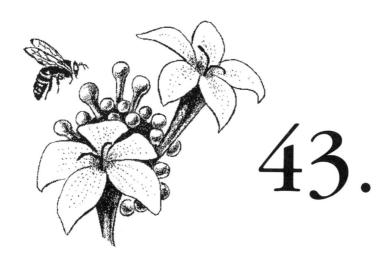

43.

THE NONI
DOUCHE

Noni fruit juice may be added to a douche bag filled with water.

USE A NONI DOUCHE
FOR CONDITIONS SUCH AS:

- Menstrual cramps.
- Vaginal itching.
- Vaginal odor.
- Yeast infections.
- Personal hygiene after intercourse.

161

How to use
A Noni Douche:

1. Fill a douche bag with warm, purified water. Add one or two ounces of Noni fruit juice to the bag. Attach the tube to the bag, and attach the applicator to the tube.

2. Find a position in the shower or bathtub that is comfortable. You may stand, squat, kneel on one knee, or lie on your back—many positions will work. You could even douche over the toilet seat.

3. Hold the douche bag above your waistline. Hold the tube lower than this, and allow any air in the tube to empty out. When the Noni-water liquid starts to come out, quickly insert the applicator into your body. Insert it as far as it will go comfortably.

4. Move the applicator as necessary to allow the liquid to cleanse the entire area. The Noni-water liquid will spill out of your body as you perform the douche.

More about
The Noni Douche:

Have a sanitary pad or panty liner ready to wear when you are finished. Any juice that leaks out could stain your clothing or the bathroom carpet.

Symptoms can be alleviated seconds after douching, though sometimes it takes a few hours to feel relief. For more stubborn or serious cases, try the Noni Vaginal Implant (page 195).

For menstrual cramps and other symptoms of PMS, try the Procedure for Chronic Conditions (page 37). Do the Noni Douche daily starting two weeks before you expect menstruation to begin.

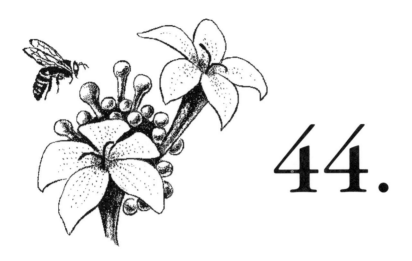

44.

NONI

EAR DROPS

Noni Ear Drops are effective for children and adults, as well as for pets.

TRY NONI EAR DROPS
FOR CONDITIONS SUCH AS:

- Chronic dizzy spells.
- Ear infections.
- Ear pain.
- Headaches.
- Impaired hearing.
- Loss of hearing.

How to Apply
Noni Ear Drops
Method 1:

1. Fill a clean glass eyedropper with Noni fruit juice.

2. Hold the eyedropper under hot water to warm the juice.

3. Put a drop of the warmed Noni on the back of your hand to test its temperature. If the Noni is still too cold, put the dropper back under the hot water. If the Noni feels too hot, wait a minute while the air temperature cools it off, then retest.

4. Have the person who is to receive the Noni Ear Drops lie on the bed facing sideways. Place a towel on the pillow, as any Noni that may leak out of the ear will stain the bed linens.

5. Apply the Noni Ear Drops.

    • For children: Place two or three drops of warm Noni fruit juice inside the ear.

    • For adults: Keep adding drops until the ear canal is filled with juice.

6. With your fingertip, gently rub behind the ear and just underneath it, to work the juice towards the eardrum.

7. Pack the ear with a small piece of cotton.

8. Repeat Steps 5, 6 and 7 with the other ear.

How to Apply
Noni Ear Drops
Method 2

Methods 2 and 3 can be used if you don't have an eyedropper. Method 2 works best if you are applying Noni Ear Drops into your own ears.

1. Warm about two teaspoonfuls of Noni fruit juice as described in the information box below.

2. Soak the end of a Q-tip in the warm Noni. Touch this wet end of the Q-tip against your cheek to check the Noni's temperature.

3. If you are applying the Noni Ear Drops to yourself, lie on your side and drape a towel over your neck and behind your ear. Press the wet end of the Q-tip against the opening of your ear canal. This will cause some of the Noni to drip into your ear. You may have to dip the Q-tip back in the Noni and repeat this step a few times until your ear is filled.

   If you are using this method on someone else, simply hold the Q-tip over the ear canal's opening. Then squeeze the cotton tip to release the juice into the ear.

4. Use the other side of the Q-tip to wipe up any Noni on the outer ear that didn't make it into the ear canal.

5. With your fingertip, gently rub behind the ear and just underneath it, to work the juice towards the eardrum.

6. Pack the ear with a piece of cotton.

7. Repeat this procedure for the other ear, using a new Q-tip.

How to Warm Noni
Ear Drops for Methods 2 and 3

1. Heat a glass or ceramic teacup by filling it with boiling water or very hot tap water.

2. After about fifteen seconds, pour out the water. The cup should be very hot.

3. Quickly dry the cup and pour in a couple teaspoonfuls of Noni fruit juice.

4. Apply the Noni immediately, before the juice cools.

How to Apply
Noni Ear Drops
Method 3:

Do not use this method with children because of the small size of their ears.

1. Warm about two teaspoonfuls of Noni fruit juice as described in the information box on the previous page.

2. Tear apart a cotton ball to make two pieces the right size to plug the opening of each ear.

3. Dip one cotton ball into the warmed Noni fruit juice so that half of it is wet. Touch the wet cotton to your cheek to check its temperature.

4. Lie on your side and hold the wet cotton over your ear canal. The wet side of the cotton should be facing your body. Squeeze the juice into your ear.

5. Then pack the same piece of cotton gently inside your ear, with the wet side facing in.

6. With your fingertip, gently rub behind your ear and just underneath it, to work the juice towards the eardrum.

7. Repeat Steps 3 through 6 with your other ear.

More about
Noni Ear Drops:

Noni Ear Drops may be applied two or three times a day.

Before pouring Noni fruit juice for Noni Ear Drops, gently turn the Noni bottle upside-down then right side up a few times. A nice mix of the pulpier part and the watery part of the Noni makes the best Noni Ear Drops. Don't shake the Noni bottle so much that air bubbles form. The ear is a relatively small area. Air bubbles in the Ear Drops would prevent the Noni from reaching all of the ear.

Massage any unused Noni Ear Drops onto swollen glands.

Our family has enjoyed relief from minor ear infections after only one or two treatments. (This was verified by examining the ears with an otoscope.) Several treatments may be necessary for more serious conditions.

Chronic ear conditions may require Noni Ear Drop treatments daily for several weeks. Meanwhile, follow the Procedure for Chronic Conditions (page 37).

For acute ear conditions, also follow the Procedure for Acute Conditions (page 35).

If an ear condition is painful, apply Noni Ear Drops and then apply a Noni Compress (page 89). One way to do this is to use a thin compress pad that is about four inches square. Gently press the Noni-soaked compress pad around the ear so it conforms to the contours of the ear. Another option is to apply a small Noni-soaked cotton ball in the indentation behind the earlobe. Apply the Noni Ear Drops daily for a few days, even after the pain subsides.

If a physician examines your ears after you have put Noni Ear Drops in them, let the doctor know that you have used Noni. The ear canal may contain purple remnants of Noni pulp. Sometimes, however, there is no trace of having used Noni in the ear. The ear seems to have eagerly absorbed the Noni, purple and all.

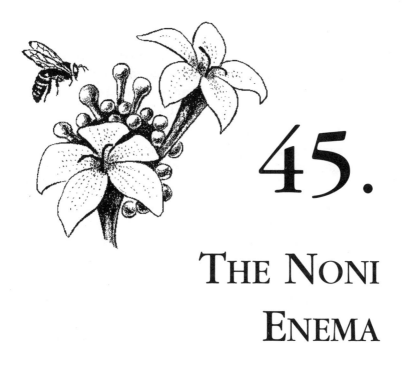

45.

THE NONI ENEMA

A relatively small amount of Noni fruit juice in an enema bag can make a big difference.

TRY A NONI ENEMA
FOR CONDITIONS SUCH AS:

- Constipation.
- Detoxification.
- Heavy metal poisoning.
- Inflammation.
- Parasites.

How to take
A Noni Enema:

1. Add warm water to a standard, two-quart enema bag until it is nearly full. If your tap water is chlorinated, use heated purified water. Test the temperature of the water in the bag with your finger to make sure it isn't too hot.

2. Add one tablespoonful of Noni fruit juice to the enema bag. If you are taking a series of enemas, gradually increase this amount. You could use up to eight ounces (one cup) of Noni per enema bag.

3. Attach the enema tube to the bag, and the enema applicator to the tube. Lubricate the applicator with an herbal ointment. Don't use a mentholated ointment—it will sting!

4. Hold the enema bag over the sink, and allow any air trapped in the bag to exit through the tube. When Noni-water liquid starts to come out of the bag, squeeze the stopper that is attached to the tube. This will stop the flow of the liquid.

5. Hook the enema bag onto a shower door or the bathroom door handle. Place an old towel on the bathroom floor. Find a comfortable position on the floor. I prefer to lie on one side. You could also lean over on your hands and knees.

6. Insert the applicator into your body. Release the stopper that is attached to the tube. Try to relax, to allow the liquid to enter your intestines. Squeeze the stopper as needed to regulate the flow of the Noni-water liquid into your body.

7. When you feel an urge to expel the liquid, squeeze the stopper and remove the applicator from your body. Try to retain the liquid for a few minutes. If the urge passes, and if you were able to successfully retain the liquid, try massaging your lower abdomen. This will help break up any accumulation in your intestines. Massage in the direction that food usually goes when passing through the intestines—looking down at your abdomen, this would be in a clockwise circle. Insert more Noni-water when you can.

8. When you are ready, expel the enema into the toilet. Some people are able to retain the entire contents of the enema bag. Others can only retain a portion of the enema at a time.

MORE ABOUT
THE NONI ENEMA:

Noni fruit juice added to an enema can help the intestines feel soothed and peaceful, despite the relative stress of the enema itself.

If your colon is very unhealthy, think twice about filling the enema bag a second time, and doing an enema immediately following the first. It may be too much activity for the intestines at one time.

Experiment with different amounts of Noni in the enema bag. This way you can find an amount that suits you best.

You may add Noni along with other natural substances that are sometimes included in enemas, such as sea-salt and liquid chlorophyll.

You may find parasites expelled into the toilet bowl, but microscopic parasites may also be eliminated, which you won't be able to see.

Here are guidelines for how often to take the Noni Enema:

1. Take the enema once a day for a week.

2. Then take the enema every other day for a couple of weeks.

3. Gradually decrease the frequency of the enemas to once a week.

If symptoms recur, repeat this schedule.

Adjust these suggestions to meet your personal needs.

To help calm and stabilize the body during a detoxification crisis, take a series of enemas and decrease the amount of Noni fruit juice that you use each time. For example, the first day you might start with two ounces of Noni fruit juice in the enema bag. The second day, you might use one ounce and the third day, add only one tablespoonful.

Whereas decreasing the amount of Noni used in a series of enemas helps to slow down a cleansing reaction, increasing the amount of Noni used in each enema would intensify a detoxification.

Noni fruit juice may also be used for colonic irrigation, which is a special procedure performed by Colon Therapists. A Noni Colonic Irrigation is more thorough and effective than a Noni Enema, and reaches farther up the intestine. Add about five ounces of Noni to the colon-therapy machine (use at least two ounces, and as much as eight to ten ounces). Perform the colonic irrigation as usual. Noni fruit juice added to a colonic irrigation can help the intestines feel soothed and peaceful, despite the relative stress of the colon therapy itself.

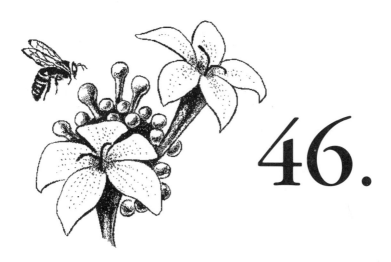

NONI EYE DROPS

Noni fruit juice may be used in the eyes. But enough water should be added to adequately disperse the Noni pulp.

USE NONI
EYE DROPS FOR:

Various conditions of the eyelid and the surface of the eye including:

- Allergic reactions that affect the eyes.

- Conjunctivitis.

- Infections.

- Inflammation.

- Itchy eyes.

- Pink-eye.

- Tear gland infections.

How to Make and
Apply Noni Eye Drops:

1. Pour a tablespoonful of Noni fruit juice in a clean cup.

2. Measure four tablespoonfuls (one-quarter cup) of purified water in a measuring cup. Pour the purified water into the Noni fruit juice in a steady, uninterrupted stream. Meanwhile, swirl the liquids together for about twenty seconds. You have now made Noni Eye Drops.

3. Fill a clean, glass eyedropper with the Noni Eye Drops.

4. Place the full eyedropper in hot tap water. This will warm the Noni-water mixture.

5. Squeeze out a drop or two of Noni Eye Drops onto the back of your hand. This serves two purposes: 1) It lets you test the temperature of the liquid. 2) It removes any tap water that might have seeped into the eyedropper while warming it.

6. Place a few drops of Noni Eye Drops in each eye.

More about
Noni Eye Drops:

Do not shake the Noni bottle before measuring juice for Noni Eye Drops. The watery portion of the juice, which tends to rise to the top of the bottle, is better for Eye Drops.

Noni Eye Drops can be applied several times a day.

As with other kinds of eye drops, the eyes may sting for a few seconds after administering the drops. A soothing feeling should follow. Interestingly, some people don't feel the sting at all, or feel it only sometimes.

Keep the Noni Eye Drops in the refrigerator. But make a fresh batch each day you plan to use them. At the end of the day, drink any unused Noni-water mixture that you may have leftover, so it won't be wasted. This oral dose can also be helpful for your eye condition.

Consider supplementing the Eye Drops treatment with a

Noni Eye Poultice (page 105). Eye Drops are especially help-ful for conditions on the surface of the eye, whereas the Eye Poultice can uplift the health of the entire eye.

For relatively serious eye conditions, also use the Proce-dure for Serious Conditions (page 41). For eye conditions that are chronic, but not so serious, also use the Procedure for Chronic Conditions (page 37).

AN ALTERNATIVE METHOD
FOR TAKING NONI EYE DROPS

If you don't like taking eye drops, you may be grateful to know there is an alternative. This is the preferred method for giving Noni Eye Drops to children. It may be easier to use this method on yourself, as well.

1. Make a Noni Eye Poultice pad as described on page 105, or simply use two cotton balls.

2. Dip the poultice pad (or cotton balls) in the Noni-water mixture that you made in Steps 1 and 2 on the previous page.

3. Place the poultice pad over your eyes. The liquid may drip off your face; so put a towel under your head.

4. Gently press the poultice pad into the inside corners of your eyes and roll your eyeballs around. This will release the Noni-water mixture into your eyes in a gentle way that you can easily control.

5. Remove the poultice pad after the eyes have been bathed in Noni. Of course, if you like, you may leave the poultice pad in place for fifteen to thirty minutes to obtain the ben-efits of a Noni Eye Poultice.

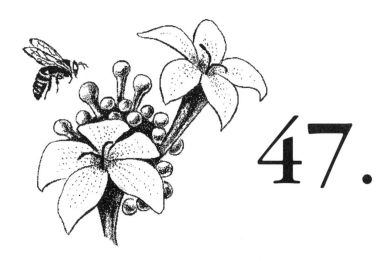

THE NONI
GARGLE

Noni's analgesic properties can alleviate a sore throat, and its antiseptic properties can fight infection.

TRY THE
NONI GARGLE FOR:

Various throat conditions including:

- Dry throat.
- Sore throat.
- Strep throat.
- Tonsillitis.
- The onset of flu-like symptoms.

How to
Gargle with Noni:

1. Take a large sip of Noni fruit juice.

2. Gargle as usual. Allow the juice to gradually drip down your throat.

3. Continue gargling until all the Noni is swallowed.

More about
The Noni Gargle:

Gargle as often as necessary throughout the day.

Gargling with warm Noni Tea (page 69) can also be soothing. But some people may prefer the feeling of gargling with cold Noni, straight from the refrigerator.

You may gargle with some or all of the daily dose of Noni that you would normally drink

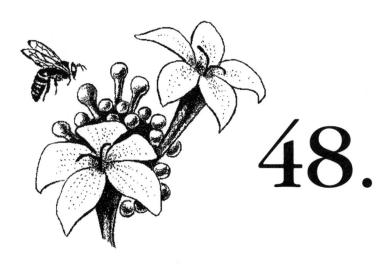

48.

NONI MOUTHWASH

A refreshing and therapeutic alternative to the mint variety.

USE NONI
MOUTHWASH FOR:

- Bad breath.
- Cancer of the mouth.
- Gingivitis.
- Gum and mouth infections.
- Mercury poisoning that affects the gums, tongue or cheeks.
- Sores on the tongue, gums, or inside the cheeks.
- Toothache.

How to use
Noni Mouthwash:

1. Take a relatively large sip of Noni fruit juice (about one-half a tablespoonful). The juice will cause you to salivate.

2. Swish the Noni-saliva mixture around your teeth and gums and every corner of your mouth. If too much saliva is produced spit out some of the liquid. Continue to swish.

   While you are swishing, you will likely have an urge to swallow. Follow your body's reflex—but without letting too much Noni drip down your throat. This really is possible, and is more easily done if you lean forward when the throat muscles contract.

3. After about a minute, the flavor of the Noni will change. This is an indication that your body has absorbed most of the Noni's healing compounds under the tongue. It is also a signal to spit out the Noni-saliva mixture.

More about
Noni Mouthwash:

Use the Noni Mouthwash two or three times daily, or as needed.

The swishing movement increases circulation, and allows the Noni to reach the entire mouth. It also incorporates air into the Noni-saliva mixture. The oxygen in this air is one of the reasons the Noni Mouthwash can make your mouth feel so good. The Noni helps carry the oxygen to the cells, oxygenating them. This in turn activates the cells, so they can receive even more of Noni's healing compounds.

You may gargle with Noni Mouthwash. If you do, it is better to gargle first, and then swish the Noni as described above.

A Noni Mouthwash can leave your teeth and gums feeling fresh and clean. It is a wonderful addition to your daily dental care routine.

If you are using the Noni Mouthwash for pain, you may feel relief immediately, or soon afterwards.

A few applications may be necessary to alleviate infection or other acute problems.

Chronic bad breath may require a daily Noni Mouthwash for a long period of time, in addition to drinking Noni every day. Try the Procedure for Chronic Conditions on page 37.

If you are using the Mouthwash for mercury poisoning, take extra care not to swallow any Noni. Also, the flavor of the Noni may change sooner for you than for most other people, so you may swish for much less than a minute. You should also rinse your mouth with purified water after you spit out the liquid.

The Noni Mouthwash may not be as intense a detoxification as the Oral Detox (page 31). The Noni Mouthwash helps draw toxins from the surface of the mouth, whereas the Oral Detox tends to draw toxins from deeper inside the tissues.

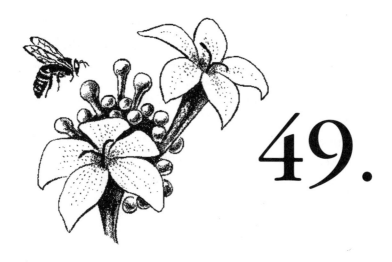

49.

NONI
NOSE DROPS

Noni Nose Drops can soothe the sinuses, reduce inflammation and ease congestion.

USE NONI NOSE DROPS
FOR CONDITIONS SUCH AS:

- Allergies that affect the sinuses.
- Colds and flu.
- Nasal infections.
- Nasal irritations.
- Sinusitis.
- Stuffy nose.

183

HOW TO MAKE
NONI NOSE DROPS:

1. Don't shake the Noni bottle before pouring Noni to make Noni Nose Drops. The watery portion of the Noni fruit juice, which tends to rise to the top of the bottle, makes better Nose Drops. Too much pulp in the Nose Drops can be mildly irritating.

2. Pour a tablespoonful of Noni fruit juice into a small, clean, glass container. Use a reclosable jar or tincture bottle.

3. Measure a tablespoonful of purified water, and pour it into the Noni in a steady, uninterrupted stream. Meanwhile, swirl the liquids together for about twenty seconds.

HOW TO APPLY NONI
NOSE DROPS
METHOD 1:

This may be the easiest method, but it requires a clean eye-dropper.

1. Fill a clean, glass eyedropper with Noni Nose Drops.

2. Hold the eyedropper in hot tap water to warm the Nose Drops.

3. Squeeze out a drop or two of Nose Drops onto the back of your hand. This serves two purposes: 1) It lets you test the temperature of the liquid. 2) It removes any tap water that might have seeped into the eyedropper while warming it.

4. Tilt your head back, or lie down. Insert a few drops of Noni Nose Drops into each nostril.

HOW TO APPLY NONI
NOSE DROPS
METHOD 2:

Use this method if you don't have an eyedropper.

Do not use this method for children because of the small size of their nostrils.

If you would like to warm the Nose Drops, use the heating method for Noni Ear Drops described in the information box on page 165.

1. Shape a piece of cotton ball into a cylinder about one inch long. It should be somewhat less wide than the diameter of your nostril's opening. Taper both ends of the cotton.

2. Saturate one end of the cotton in the Noni Nose Drops solution.

3. Tilt your head back, or lie down. Have a towel or tissue paper handy to catch any Noni Nose Drops that drip on your face.

4. Insert the wet end of the cotton inside your nostril. At least half of the cotton should remain outside your nose.

5. When you insert the cotton, some of the Noni Noni Drops will drip into your nose. To release more liquid from the cotton, gently press the side of your nose against the cotton that is inside it. You will feel the liquid drip into your sinuses.

6. Repeat this procedure for the other nostril, using a second piece of cotton.

MORE ABOUT
NONI NOSE DROPS:

Noni Nose Drops can be given as often as every few minutes to help clear and soothe the sinuses. Or, apply them a few times a day, as needed.

Remember, Noni is a purplish color and Noni Nose Drops may loosen and dissolve mucus. Don't be surprised when you blow your nose and see purple-stained mucus in the tissue paper.

Store Noni Nose Drops in the refrigerator in a reclosable glass container. The quantity of Noni Nose Drops solution suggested in the recipe on the previous page will be enough for several applications of Nose Drops. But make a fresh batch each day you plan to use them. At the end of the day, drink any unused Nose Drops that you may have leftover, so they won't be wasted.

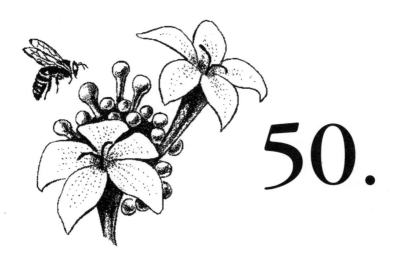

50.

THE NONI
RECTAL IMPLANT

Not a place you might expect to put a fruit juice! But if you have problems here, you'll be glad you did.

TRY THE NONI
RECTAL IMPLANT FOR:
Various conditions of the rectum and lower bowel including:

- Cancer.
- Diverticulitis.
- Fissures.
- Hemorrhoids.
- Inflammation.

187

How to do a
Noni Rectal Implant:

1. Purchase a small disposable enema bottle from the drug-store. Open the bottle and pour the prepackaged liquid down the sink. Rinse out the bottle. Pour one or two ounces of Noni fruit juice into the bottle and replace the bottle top.

2. Hold the bottle in a sink full of hot tap water to warm the Noni.

3. Lubricate the bottle tip with an herbal ointment, such as a comfrey salve. (Don't use petroleum jelly, which will prevent Noni from reaching any area that the petroleum jelly covers. And don't use an ointment that contains menthol—or it will sting.)

4. Find a comfortable position either lying on one side, lying on your back, bending over the sink, or leaning over on your hands and knees. Insert the bottle tip into your rectum. Squeeze the bottle to release the Noni into your body.

5. Hold the Noni in your body for as long as possible. Try to keep it in for at least five minutes. It is preferable to retain the Noni in your rectum until it is completely absorbed.

More about the
Noni Rectal Implant:

If you have problems of the lower bowel and rectum, it is especially important to apply Noni there directly. When you drink Noni, its healing compounds spread throughout your body. But not enough of these compounds reach the lower bowel and rectum to be therapeutic—though they will help your condition indirectly by uplifting your overall health.

Ideally, try to do the Noni Rectal Implant after you have taken an enema, or have had a bowel movement. Then your rectum will be empty. If you take an enema beforehand, add a tablespoonful of Noni to the enema bag after it has been filled with warm water. It is important to expel as much of the enema into the toilet as possible before doing the Noni Rectal Implant. If too much water remains in your body, you may have a greater-than-usual urge to expel the Implant.

If you have an urge to expel the Implant, try to keep the Implant in for at least a few minutes, then follow the urge. This urge may be your body's way of flushing toxins that the Noni has helped release.

If your body has an immediate strong urge to expel the Implant, use less Noni next time.

If the rectum is highly irritated, the Noni might burn slightly at first. But soothing relief should soon follow.

Perform the implant daily. If your condition is relatively serious, gradually increase the amount of Noni in the implant. You can use three to four ounces per treatment. (Disposable enema bottles usually hold up to four ounces of liquid.)

When symptoms subside, gradually reduce the number of times you do the implant each week.

You can reuse the disposable enema bottle if you wash the bottle and the bottle tip with soap and water.

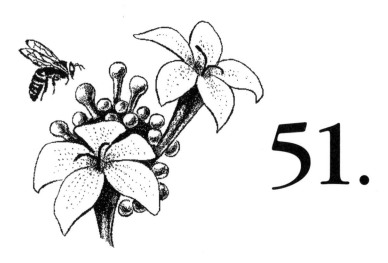

51.

THE NONI
TOOTH AND GUM
COMPRESS

The mouth and gums seem to be more sensitive to Noni's analgesic properties than most other areas of the body.

USE THE NONI TOOTH
AND GUM COMPRESS FOR:

- Gum infection.
- Helping to heal an area after dental work.
- Helping to numb an area before dental work.
- Tooth infection and toothache.

How to Make and Apply
The Noni Tooth and Gum Compress:

1. Make a Tooth and Gum Compress pad using either a cotton ball or sterile gauze. If you use cotton, form it into a cylinder about two inches long and about one-quarter inch wide. If you use gauze, roll it into a cylinder of about the same size.

2. Pour a tablespoonful of Noni fruit juice into a small bowl. Press the compress pad into the Noni. Wipe up any pulp that remains in the bowl with the pulpy side of the compress pad.

3. Insert the wet compress pad into your mouth, with the pulpy side of the pad against your skin. Press the pad above your gum line between the affected area and your cheek. It is okay to swallow any Noni fruit juice that leaks out. However the swallowing action tends to draw the Noni out of the compress. Try to avoid this as much as possible.

4. Leave the compress pad in place for ten to fifteen minutes. By then much of the Noni fruit juice in the pad will have been swallowed and replaced by saliva. Even so, the pulp that clings to the compress pad would still be working.

5. Remove the compress pad and discard it.

6. Repeat the Noni Tooth and Gum Compress as often as needed.

More about the Noni
Tooth and Gum Compress:

Even if the pain is in a small area, make the compress pad about two inches long and treat the entire portion of the jaw where the pain is located. By using a relatively large compress pad, more of Noni's healing compounds will be absorbed into the area. You will then get the most benefit possible from Noni's therapeutic and analgesic properties.

The procedure on the previous page can be used for tooth and gum conditions of all kinds. However, if you have pain from an unfilled tooth cavity, you may benefit by adding to the procedure as follows:

1. Clean out the cavity with a toothbrush.

2. Apply the Noni Tooth and Gum Compress as outlined in Steps 1, 2, and 3 above.

3. Dry the tooth with a clean cloth or piece of gauze.

4. Make a second compress pad using a piece of a cotton ball. It should be small enough to cover the affected tooth. Soak the pad in some Noni fruit juice.

5. Place this second pad over the affected tooth.

6. Press the pad on the tooth to fill the cavity with Noni. Hold this pad in place with the opposing teeth. Keep both compress pads in place for ten to fifteen minutes. By then, much of the Noni in the pad will have been swallowed or replaced by saliva.

7. Remove both compress pads and discard them. Repeat the above procedure as often as needed.

People have different levels of pain tolerance, so a Tooth and Gum Compress's analgesic effect will vary. Some people may be able to use Noni instead of painkillers during or after routine dental work. Also try taking a Trauma Dose right before dental work begins, to help you relax and to better handle the stress of dental work.

Routinely apply the Noni Tooth and Gum Compress both before and after any dental work you may receive. Doing the Compress beforehand can reduce any traumatic effects you may experience; doing it afterwards can promote healing.

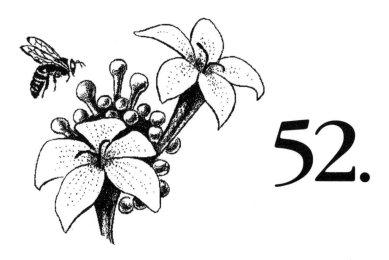

52.

THE NONI
VAGINAL IMPLANT

Noni can be implanted using a small disposable enema bottle, large plastic syringe tube—or even a turkey baster!

USE THE NONI VAGINAL IMPLANT FOR:
Various conditions of the cervix, uterus, and vagina including:

- Cervical Cancer.
- Endometriosis.
- Uterine cancer.
- Uterine prolapse.
- Vaginitis.
- Yeast infections.

HOW TO APPLY
THE NONI VAGINAL IMPLANT:

1. Gather the things you will need to do the implant.

   • A pillow for your head.

   • A rolled up bath towel or another pillow to elevate your hips. (If you use a pillow, cover it with a towel.)

   • A feminine napkin.

   • A panty-liner for afterwards.

   • A small towel for clean up.

   • Perhaps something to read to pass the time.

   Use old towels, because Noni fruit juice will stain and getting them wet is unavoidable.

2. Add Noni fruit juice to a plastic syringe tube. This is the best kind of applicator because it allows you to easily control how quickly the Noni is dispensed. The standard dose for a Noni Vaginal Implant is one ounce.

3. Lie on your back, with your hips on the pillow.

4. Put the end of the applicator inside your body and slowly insert the Noni fruit juice. With your other hand, hold the feminine napkin under the syringe, to catch any juice that spills. Try not to cough or sneeze, and try to relax your abdominal muscles. You'll soon discover how best to relax in order to retain as much of the Noni as possible.

5. After you have inserted the Noni, remain lying in this position for about 15 to 20 minutes.

6. When you are ready to get up, hold the feminine napkin and the small towel between your legs to catch the juice. Most of it will spill out when you rise.

7. Wear the panty-liner to collect any remaining Noni that may leak out later.

MORE ABOUT THE
NONI VAGINAL IMPLANT:

The Noni Vaginal Implant is usually performed once a day. However, consider doing the Implant twice a day if it causes vaginal detoxification accompanied by foul odor, mucus discharge, or tissue sloughing.

Plastic syringe tubes are the easiest applicators to use. They can be purchased at pet stores, especially those that specialize in large birds. (They are intended for hand-feeding large baby parrots.)

Find a syringe that holds two ounces of liquid. The plunger in a one-ounce syringe tends to fall out easily when the syringe contains a full ounce of liquid. If you use a one-ounce syringe because that's all you can find, fill it twice using half an ounce of liquid each time.

You may not need to warm the juice as you would for Noni Ear Drops or Eye Drops, because the vaginal tissue is less sensitive to temperature.

It may be more convenient to do the Vaginal Implant when you are in bed for the night. Just keep your bed linens well protected.

If you have a prolapse, it will be difficult to implant much juice at first. Start with one-half ounce of Noni and work up to an ounce as the condition improves. Even if you use only one-half ounce of Noni, you may be able to insert only a small portion of this at a time. Hold as much of it inside you as you can; though it may leak right out, just insert a little more. Do this until the entire half once of Noni has been used.

Though the Noni used in the Vaginal Implant won't come into direct contact with the ovaries, the Vaginal Implant can still be helpful for ovarian conditions. The Vaginal Implant will help uplift the health of the entire female reproductive system, which includes the ovaries, and may provide a pathway for toxins in the ovaries to leave the body.

Because the Implant uplifts the health of the entire area, the Implant can also be helpful for endometriosis. For this condition, also apply a Noni Poultice (page 93) over the areas of pain.

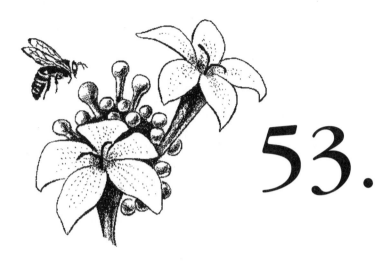

THE NONI
VAGINAL WIPE

A fast and easy way to alleviate minor discomforts.

WHEN TO USE
THE NONI VAGINAL WIPE:

- After childbirth.
- For vaginal itching.
- For mild yeast infections.
- To freshen up after intercourse.
- To soothe chapped, irritated or dry labia.

How to Apply
The Noni Vaginal Wipe:

1. Dip a cotton ball in Noni fruit juice, so that only half of it gets wet.

2. Wipe the wet side of the cotton ball inside the vaginal opening. Then wipe between the labia. Squeeze the cotton ball as you apply it, or press it against your body, to release the Noni onto your skin.

More about the
Noni Vaginal Wipe:

This procedure can be done after every urination, or as needed.

Press the wet cotton against particularly sore or itchy areas to release the juice directly onto those areas.

Relief may come on contact with the Noni, or several minutes later. Several applications may be needed. For more serious conditions, apply a Noni Compress (page 89) over the area or try a Noni Vaginal Implant (page 195).

After childbirth, your labia may be too tender to apply Noni with a cotton ball. Instead, add a tablespoonful or more of Noni to a sani-bottle that has been filled with warm water. After urination, squirt the Noni-water mixture onto your labia. This can feel especially soothing.

APPENDIX A

HEALTH
EVALUATION SHEETS

Healing is a natural function of the body. It is also natural to forget we ever had certain symptoms once they've gone away. This questionnaire will help you remember the symptoms you used to have, so you can better appreciate the difference in how you feel now.

USE THESE HEALTH
EVALUATION SHEETS FOR:

- Keeping track of your health progress.
- Evaluating how well Noni has helped you.
- Evaluating the effectiveness of certain Noni dosages and applications.

(cont.)

201

- Your personal testimony to the effects of Noni, which you can keep confidential, or share with your doctor, or your family, friends and associates.

HOW TO USE THESE
HEALTH EVALUATION SHEETS:

1. Complete Part 1 before you start taking Noni fruit juice (or as soon as possible thereafter). Give brief, honest answers. When you have finished Part 1, don't look at what you've written until after you have completed Part 2.

2. Make some copies of Part 2.*

3. After taking Noni daily for about a month or two, complete a copy of Part 2.

4. Compare your answers on Part 2, with what you wrote earlier on Part 1. Use a marking pen to highlight those answers that are significantly different.

5. A few months later, complete another copy of Part 2. Compare your answers with those you gave on evaluation sheets you had previously completed. Use what you learn from these evaluation sheets to adjust how you are using Noni.

6. From time to time, monitor your health progress by completing another copy of Part 2.

* Permission has been granted from the copyright holder.

Health Evaluation Sheet - Part 1

Please complete the following sentences before you start to take Noni, or as soon as possible thereafter:

Overall, my health is _____

The five parts of my body, which bother me the most (in order) are: 1) _____
2) _____ 3) _____ 4) _____ 5) _____

These areas have bothered me for this length of time: 1) _____ 2) _____ 3) _____ 4) _____ 5) _____

I would describe my worst pain as _____

When I wake up in the morning, my pain is _____

When it's bedtime, my pain is _____

After I eat, my body feels _____

My bowel and bladder regularity is _____

My menstrual cycles are _____

My libido is _____

My skin feels _____

My hands feel _____

My feet feel _____

My joints feel _____

My circulation is _____

My body weight seems _____

In general, my emotions are _____

My mental clarity and memory is _____

I am taking Noni fruit juice for _____

I think Noni fruit juice will _____

The one thing I would like most to change about my health is _____

Health Evaluation Sheet - Part 2

Please complete the following sentences after you have taken Noni for a while:

Overall, my health is _____

The five parts of my body, which bother me the most (in order) are: 1) _____
2) _____ 3) _____ 4) _____ 5) _____

These areas have bothered me for this length of time: 1) _____ 2) _____ 3) _____ 4) _____ 5) _____

I would describe my worst pain as _____

When I wake up in the morning, my pain is _____

When it's bedtime, my pain is _____

After I eat, my body feels _____

My bowel and bladder regularity is _____

My menstrual cycles are _____

My libido is _____

My skin feels _____

My hands feel _____

My feet feel _____

My joints feel _____

My circulation is _____

My body weight seems _____

In general, my emotions are _____

My mental clarity and memory is _____

I am taking Noni fruit juice for _____

I think Noni fruit juice will _____

The one thing I would like most to change about my health is _____

APPENDIX B

CLEANSING REACTIONS

The body is naturally cleansing itself of toxins and metabolic wastes all the time. A cleansing reaction (also called a healing crisis or detoxification crisis) may occur when something that promotes good health, like Noni fruit juice, helps your body release more toxins than your organs can handle at once.

COMMON CLEANSING REACTIONS INCLUDE:

- Bad breath or body odor.
- Boils and pimples.
- Cough.
- Diarrhea or loose stools.
  (cont.)

- Emotional releases.
- Foul smelling urine.
- Headaches.
- Heavier than usual bleeding at menstruation.
- Intestinal gas or bloating.
- Joint pain due to release of uric acid crystals.
- Mucus discharge.
- Skin rashes.
- Swollen glands.
- Unusual fatigue.

How do I know if I'm Having a Cleansing Reaction?

Sometimes it can indeed be difficult to know the difference between a cleansing reaction, an allergic reaction, or hypersensitivity to Noni's healing compounds.

If you get a reaction <u>immediately</u> after taking Noni:

- You may have an allergy to Noni.

  Suspect that this is the case if your symptoms include your body's typical responses to things you are allergic to. Wait until your symptoms subside. Then try the Noni Tummy Treatment (page 151). The skin may be an effective barrier to your allergic reaction, while also allowing you to receive the benefits of Noni's healing compounds.

  If the Tummy Treatment gives you a rash, or you get another sign of an allergy, you probably are allergic to Noni. It may be best not to take Noni at this time.

- You might be hypersensitive to Noni's healing compounds.

  Suspect that this is the case if your symptoms do not include your body's typical responses to things you are allergic to. Wait until your symptoms subside. Then try the

Noni Tummy Treatment (page 151). The Tummy Treatment can help your body adjust gradually to Noni. If you do not get a rash or any other cleansing reaction, continue the topical application daily. Give your body time to become accustomed to Noni. Use the Procedure for Gradually Introducing Noni to the Body (page 53).

- You may be having an immediate cleansing reaction.

  Suspect that this is the case if:

  - Your symptoms include foul odors, and are unlike your body's typical responses to things you are allergic to.

  - Your body was already primed for a cleansing, and Noni just provided the supportive boost needed to proceed.

  - You have been drinking less than two glasses of water a day and toxins have been building up in your body.

    Make sure you are drinking at least eight glasses of purified water a day, to flush the metabolic wastes your body naturally produces, plus the toxins your body collects from your diet and from the environment. If you have not been drinking enough water and you get a cleansing reaction, your symptoms can go away if you simply drink more water.

  The following day, try another dose of Noni. If the Noni eases your symptoms, you have likely had an immediate cleansing reaction. Continue to take Noni to assist your body through the cleanse.

If you have been taking Noni for a while, and then get cleansing symptoms:

- You are probably not allergic to Noni or hypersensitive to Noni's healing compounds, since you have been taking Noni for a while without having had a reaction.

- You may be experiencing either a cleansing reaction or the flu. It can be hard to know which is which because:

- Both cleansing reactions and the flu tend to last the same amount of time. Both can be acute and short-lived; however, both can also drag out for quite a while.

- Natural methods for enhancing the immune system will help in either case.

- Antibiotics, cough-suppressants, and other pharmaceutical medicines often suppress a cleansing reaction. But they may be necessary in some cases to stabilize the body, so it can gain strength for a more gradual detoxification later.

> Please see a Health Professional if your symptoms become more than you can comfortably address with home remedies.

You probably have a cold or flu if:

If you have been taking a Maintenance Dose (page 11) of one ounce daily. Generally, one ounce a day of Noni is enough to supply the body's daily need for Noni's healing compounds. It is unlikely that this much Noni would initiate a cleansing reaction in most people.

You are probably having a cleansing reaction if:

You are doing or have recently done:

- The Top Dose Procedure.

- A Noni Fast.

- The Technique for Stubborn Conditions.

WHAT TO DO IF YOU THINK
YOU ARE HAVING A CLEANSING REACTION:

Here are some ways you can use Noni to ease your cleansing symptoms if you think you may be having a cleansing reaction:

- Make sure you drink at least eight glasses of purified water a day. Water is essential to help flush toxins out of the system.

- Substitute a dose of Noni Tea (page 69) for each dose of Noni that you usually take.

- Drink an extra dose or two of Noni, in the form of Noni Tea.

- Try taking the same number of doses as usual, but take only about half a tablespoonful each time as an Auto-dilution (page 27).

- Use the Noni Tummy Treatment either in place of your regular Noni doses, or in addition to them.

- Try drinking a half a glass of water both before and after taking a dose of Noni. This will encourage Noni's healing compounds to enter your body more gradually—with less immediate impact. Those who feel their body is particularly toxic may try this technique with every dose of Noni that they take, in order to encourage a more gradual detoxification.

- Try the Noni Fast Method 2 (page 65).

- Combine Noni fruit juice with other modalities. Noni is compatible with all natural healing methods including: herbs, homeopathic remedies, chiropractic, Chinese Medicine, Ayurvedic Medicine, Bach flower essences, vitamins and minerals, chelation therapy, acupuncture, massage, and others.

POSITIVE
CLEANSING REACTIONS:

Although cleansing reactions have a reputation for being associated with unpleasant symptoms, they can also be positive. Unfortunately, positive cleansing reactions don't last as long as we might like them to. Positive reactions include:

- A profound ability to see the overview of life itself, or of various situations that we may be involved with.

- A surge of creativity and new ideas.

- An extraordinary sense of well being.

- An unusual clarity and insight into the meaning of one's life.

- Considerably more energy than usual.

- Dreams which are easier to remember, more profound, and more meaningful.

- Greatly improved memory.

- Remarkably clearer thinking.

- Unusual hypersensitivity to one's own thoughts, needs and feelings, as well as to those of others.

Naturally, we welcome the positive cleansing reactions, but try not to be disappointed when they go away. Your body will soon adjust to the greater level of health, and the positive reactions will lessen as you settle into a new, healthier state of "normal". Continue to take Noni to help maintain this higher level of health.

MORE ABOUT
CLEANSING REACTIONS

Old injuries and health challenges, and particularly intense emotions may also surface briefly. These too are a kind of cleansing reaction. Old injuries and conditions tend to arise in reverse order, as progressively older conditions are re-experienced and then pass away. Be sure to address them with the appropriate topical and internal Noni applications, in addition to you daily oral doses of Noni.

Loose stools tend to occur when you are taking more Noni than you need. This may occur, for example, if you are a nursing mother taking extra Noni for a sick baby. The Noni you drink will pass into your breastmilk. You will have to weigh the benefits of the Noni for your baby against the relative inconvenience of frequent visits to the bathroom.

Ideally, using Noni should allow you to detoxify gradually and feel good at the same time. Then, if you do have a cleansing reaction, adjusting the amount of Noni you take and how you take it can help you detoxify more comfortably.

> In general, any reaction to Noni is better than no reaction at all. The reaction proves that your body recognizes Noni and that Noni can indeed affect you. Now the goal is to figure out what amounts, dosages and applications of Noni your body needs to function at its best.

Appendix C

What if Noni Doesn't Seem to Work for Me?

If Noni doesn't seem to be helping or isn't working as fast as you would like, ask yourself the following questions. The answers may help you understand what may be happening, and give you some ideas about what to do.

For what condition are you taking Noni?
It helps to decide why you are taking Noni. This makes it easier to correlate Noni's effects with changes in your health.

How long have you had this condition?
If your condition is chronic and long-standing, you may need more time on any health improvement program before you see results. In the process of healing, healthier cells replace sick or damaged cells. This always seems to take longer than

one would like. You probably won't feel a difference in your health until enough of these replacements have been made.

How long have you been taking Noni?
In some cases, it can take several months before you may enjoy positive changes in your health. Give Noni a fair chance to work, and give yourself a fair opportunity to heal.

How much Noni fruit juice are you taking?
Some people's bodies need more Noni than others do, even for maintenance. In general, the more serious the condition the more Noni you may need.

Are you taking Noni fruit juice regularly?
When addressing any health condition with Noni fruit juice, it is important to take your doses regularly, and without interruption. Make sure you have enough juice on hand so you won't run out.

Have you filled out Part 1 of the Health Evaluation Sheets, in Appendix A?
If you have, maybe now is the time to fill out the second sheet (Part 2) and compare your health then and now.

If you have not filled out the sheet, try to remember what your condition was like before you started to take Noni. Write down what symptoms you had. How severe were they? Take an honest look at how you feel now. Is there any difference at all?

Ask a friend or family member to recall your state of health and well being before you began taking Noni, and to evaluate your health as it is now. This feedback will be invaluable. It may be more helpful than your own evaluation, in deciding how well Noni is working for you.

HAVE YOU NOTICED ANY UNEXPECTED CHANGES IN YOUR HEALTH?

Have you noticed any improvement in minor discomforts? It is easy to overlook these kinds of improvements, especially if you are taking Noni for a major health challenge. (For example, I had no idea my eyesight had improved until someone mentioned that theirs had. I may never have noticed otherwise. I also thought that having a small amount of vaginal discharge daily was normal—until it went away after taking Noni!)

HAVE YOU HAD ANY CLEANSING REACTIONS SINCE YOU STARTED TAKING NONI?

For a list of common cleansing reactions, see pages 209-210. Cleansing reactions, though generally uncomfortable, should be considered beneficial because they signal that the body is experiencing a major cleansing. Detoxification is often a necessary first step before cell repair and health building can begin.

DID NONI EVER WORK FOR YOU AT ALL?

There is a difference between the experience of not ever having noticed any effects from Noni at all, either positive or negative, and the experience of noticing a difference at first, and then nothing thereafter.

If you have never, ever noticed anything from Noni, and you have been taking Noni for at least a few months, then perhaps your body simply doesn't need Noni's healing compounds. Or maybe your body doesn't know how to put these compounds to good use.

If you noticed a difference at first, and then nothing since, you know that Noni can help you. It may now be working below the threshold of your ability to perceive its effects. Or, it may be helping you to maintain your present level of health, and preventing it from getting worse.

Try increasing your daily dose of Noni. You might also try the Top Dose Procedure (page 15), the Procedure for Stubborn Conditions (page 49), or one of the Noni Fasts (pages 61 and 65).

What about positive changes in your personality, emotions, mental clarity, or memory?

Sometimes Noni seems to work on our non-physical aspects first. We may become more patient, calm, joyful, better able to handle stress and emotions, or perhaps less irritable, impatient or moody. Don't overlook these possible health benefits as well.

Are you taking other health supplements?

Noni is not a cure-all. Although Noni provides important micronutrients, it does not supply all the micronutrients that the body needs. It is possible that your condition would benefit from other supplements. Try a full-spectrum vitamin and mineral supplement, which would help meet all your nutrient requirements.

What activities do you now enjoy since you began to take Noni?

Sometimes the best gauge of improved health is not how we feel, but how well we can enjoy life.

APPENDIX D

WHAT IF MY SYMPTOMS RETURN?

Some people find that after Noni alleviates certain symptoms, these symptoms eventually return. It is tempting to say that Noni has stopped working. But this is not necessarily the case. Here are a few possible explanations, plus some ideas for how you can use Noni if your symptoms do come back.

• Many people who start taking Noni say they feel better almost right away. They may be experiencing positive cleansing reactions (page 214), which may be making them feel so good, they don't notice their symptoms. Unfortunately, their symptoms will probably "return" when the positive cleansing reactions no longer mask them. Lasting positive changes in one's health won't occur until they are supported by actual changes in the cells. These changes usually take time.

- After taking Noni, many people find they can eat foods that once before caused certain symptoms such as indigestion, headaches or joint pain. They find they can work harder, play harder, go to bed later and get up earlier, too.

  Instead of using Noni's healing compounds to help us grow healthier, we often use them to help us get away with doing things that are stressful (albeit enjoyable). There is nothing wrong with this. But if we abuse the freedom, it won't last.

  When the body can no longer handle the added stress, we will again need more sleep, and favorite foods will again cause discomfort. Symptoms may appear to return, when really they weren't given the opportunity to heal in the first place.

- The body will continue to age and manifest stress at its weakest points, no matter how wonderful are the therapies that we give to it. If new stresses are introduced into our lives, these weakest points may again reveal themselves and conditions that were once alleviated may return.

- During the healing process, pain and other symptoms may go away. But this doesn't mean our ailment is cured. It can take a while for healthy cells to replace unhealthy cells. Meanwhile, we may become more active than before, and cause additional stress on the healing tissue. Symptoms may return, simply to remind us to take better care of ourselves.

- Health improves in cycles: A period of health building follows every period of well being. This health-building period may pass unnoticed or make us feel more tired than usual. Or it may include an intense cleansing, when the body releases toxins, wastes, fat, and various excesses that it may have been storing. As these toxins enter the bloodstream, they pass by our weak or problem areas. These toxins can irritate these areas, causing symptoms to temporarily resurface or get worse.

- Symptoms can be signals to take better care of ourselves. Recurring symptoms may be our body's best way to tell us we need something that we have not yet given to our body. Perhaps we need more rest, or a nutrient that is missing from our diet.

- Recurring symptoms may also alert us to look at our condition from another angle. Perhaps there are mental or emotional causes that we have been overlooking. Sometimes physical improvement cannot continue until we take care of the mental and emotional aspects of ourselves.

- Dr. Ralph Heinicke offered yet another explanation for why symptoms may return, in a letter he wrote to me in October, 1997. He writes, "I now believe that some people have a marginal supply of several crucial micronutrients. Initially proxeronine is the limiting factor. This explains the tremendous response [from taking Noni], which some people observe. However, after taking Noni for a while, other micronutrients become limiting factors for good health."

  Dr. Heinicke then offers two approaches, "1) to discover what the next specific health limiting factor is, or 2) to take a supplement which contains a wide variety of potentially limiting factors."

Returning symptoms often go away again after Interrupting Noni Therapy (page 19) for a few days. In fact, after resuming Noni, health sometimes takes a leap for the better.

Here are some ideas that may explain why Interrupting Noni Therapy works:

- Symptoms may return if the body becomes accustomed to Noni's healing compounds. To obtain the same results as before, the body would need greater amounts of Noni. Taking larger doses may indeed help—for a while.

Interrupting Noni Therapy seems to readjust the body's relationship to Noni's healing compounds. Then, the smaller, and/or previous dosages of Noni become helpful once again.

- The cells in our body are innately intelligent, and like us, they have a memory and can take on both good and bad habits. As new cells replace old cells, the new cells may not know what conditions were once like without Noni. They may take the now-constant supply of Noni's healing compounds for granted and not use them as best they could. Interrupting Noni Therapy encourages the cells to use these compounds more effectively and efficiently.

- Another possibility is that when certain unused Noni compounds are stored in the body for too long, they may start to cause stress. Perhaps they deteriorate into other compounds. If this is so, maybe Interrupting Noni Therapy clears out the old stores. Then Noni usually works just as well, if not better, than it did before.

If your symptoms return, but it is not appropriate to Interrupt Noni Therapy because you have immune deficiency conditions, diabetes, cancer, or a life-threatening condition, here are some techniques you could try:

- Take sips of your doses on a regular time schedule. For example, take a sip every five, fifteen or sixty minutes. Set a timer to ensure you keep to the rhythm.

- Try the Auto-dilution (page 27) and the Noni Tummy Treatment (page 151). Also try other topical and internal Noni applications that are appropriate for your condition.

- Try Sipping (page 23) your doses of Noni if you usually drink them All at Once (page 25). Or, try drinking them All at Once if you usually Sip them.

- Examine your diet and lifestyle. Are you taking part in any activities that might be stressing your body? Find out what foods you may be allergic to, and eliminate them from your diet. Some Health Practitioners have ways to test for allergies, which can give you immediate feedback. Get more rest, try meditation or spiritual exercise, and take better care of yourself emotionally, mentally and physically.

ENDNOTES

1 Neil Solomon, M.D., Ph. D., *Liquid Island Noni* (Pleasant Grove; Woodland Publishing, 1998), p.25.

2 *Noni—Polynesia's Natural Pharmacy* (Vineyard: Pride Publishing, 1997), pp. 17,18.

3 Julia Morton, "The Ocean-Going Noni, or Indian Mulberry and Some of Its Colorful Relatives," *Economic Botany*, Vol. 46 (3), 1992.

4 Chafique Younos, Alain Rolland, Jacques Fleurentin, Marie-Claire Lanhers, Rene Misslin, and Francois Mortier, "Analgesic and Behavioural Effects of *Morinda citrifolia*," *Planta Med,* Vol. 56, 1990.

5 Tomonori Hiramatsu, Masaya Imoto, Takashi Koyano, Kazuo Umezawa, "Induction of Normal Phenotypes in *Ras*-Transformed Cells by Damnacanthal from *Morinda citrifolia*," *Cancer Letters*, Vol. 73, 1993.

6 R. M. Heinicke, "The Pharmacologically Active Ingredient of Noni," University of Hawaii. (Http://www.hookele.com /noni/active.html.)

7 Fleur L. Strand, *Physiology: A Regulatory Systems Approach*, (New York: Macmillan, 1978), pp. 31, 56, 57, 63.

8   R. M. Heinicke, "The Pharmacologically Active Ingredient of Noni."

9   *Noni—Polynesia's Natural Pharmacy*, (Vineyard: Pride Publishing, 1997), 500 South Geneva Road, Vineyard, UT, 84058. 1-800-748-2996

10 Rita Elkins M.H., "Noni (*Morinda citrifolia*) Prize Herb of the South Pacific" (Pleasant Grove: Woodland Publishing, 1997), P.O. Box 160, Pleasant Grove, UT 84062.

11 Dr. Ralph Heinicke, *"Cell Regeneration: Unlocking the Secrets of Tahitian Noni"*, audiocassette, copyright ©1996 Morinda™, Inc.

12 Notes taken during a Question and Answer period featuring Dr. Ralph Heinicke, at the 1997 Morinda™, Inc. Conference, August 12, 1997. Las Vegas, Nevada.

13 *American Red Cross: Community First Aid & Safety*, (St Louis: Mosby Lifeline, 1993), p. 147.

14 ibid.

15 ibid.

16 ibid.

17 ibid.

18 ibid.

19 *Reader's Digest Action Guide: What to do in an Emergency*, pp. 7-9.

20 *American Red Cross: Community First Aid & Safety*, p. 147.

21 Dr. Ralph Heinicke, *"Cell Regeneration: Unlocking the Secrets of Tahitian Noni"*, audiocassette, copyright ©1996 Morinda™, Inc.

INDEX

A

Abdominal conditions 152
Ability to see the overview of life
   214
Abrasions 118
Abscesses 147
Accidents 58
Acne 109, 139, 141, 149
Acupuncture 213
Acute Conditions 23
   definition of 23, 35
   Procedure for 35-37
   serious 42
Acute pain 23
Addictions 13, 41, 58
Addictive substances
   overcoming cravings for 23, 31
Adrenal conditions 94
After-shave 110
   Procedure for 99-100
Aging 37, 222
   skin 109
Air bubbles in Noni fruit juice 166
Alcohol 58
Alertness, increased 29
Allergic reactions 149

verses cleansing reactions 10
Allergies 37, 173, 183, 225
Allergy to Noni 5, 10, 54, 210
   Tummy Treatment for 152
Amalgam fillings 29
Analgesic effects 177, 103, 193
Anger 58
Ankles 124, 125
Anti-acid Substitute 73,
   159-161
Anti-inflammatory agent 8
Antibiotics 212
Antiseptic properties 177
Appetite, Noni's effect on 29
Arthritis 37, 113, 123, 127
Asthma 37, 93
Athlete's foot 39, 123
Athletic injuries 42, 89
   speeding recovery time 83
Athletic performance 83
Auto-Dilution 27-31
   verses Oral Detox 33
Auto-dilution 224
   to ease cleansing reactions 213
Auto-immune conditions 21, 27, 42

229

235

237

239

NOTE FROM THE PUBLISHER

We hope you enjoyed *53 Ways to Use Noni Fruit Juice*. If you have had success with the procedures described, or have suggestions on new techniques or different ways to use the techniques presented in this book, we would love to hear from you. We are especially interested in stories of how pregnant woman have used Noni fruit juice, and how parents have used it with their children. Please write: Pride Publishing, 500 South Geneva Road, Vineyard, Utah 84058.

If you have correspondence for the author, we would be happy to forward it to her. But keep in mind that Isabelle Navarre-Brown is not a physician, and cannot prescribe treatment or provide medical advice of any kind.